CHANGING SEXUALITIES AND PARENTAL FUNCTIONS IN THE TWENTY-FIRST CENTURY

Psychoanalysis & Women Series
Series Editor: Frances Thomson-Salo

Feminine Sensuality
Alcira Mariam Alizade

The Embodied Female
Edited by Alcira Mariam Alizade

Studies on Femininity
Edited by Alcira Mariam Alizade

Masculine Scenarios
Edited by Alcira Mariam Alizade

On Incest: Psychoanalytic Perspectives
Edited by Giovanna Ambrosio

Motherhood in the Twenty-First Century
Edited by Alcira Mariam Alizade

Masculinity and Femininity Today
Edited by Ester Palerm Marí and Frances Thomson-Salo

Women and Creativity: A Psychoanalytic Glimpse through Art, Literature, and Social Structure
Edited by Laura Tognoli Pasquali and Frances Thomson-Salo

Homosexualities: Psychogenesis, Polymorphism, and Countertransference
Edited by Elda Abrevaya and Frances Thomson-Salo

Myths of Mighty Women: Their Application in Psychoanalytic Psychotherapy
Edited by Arlene Kramer Richards and Lucille Spira

Medea: Myth and Unconscious Fantasy
Edited by Esa Roos

The Status of Women: Violence, Identity, and Activism
Edited by Vivian B. Pender

CHANGING SEXUALITIES AND PARENTAL FUNCTIONS IN THE TWENTY-FIRST CENTURY

edited by

Cândida Sé Holovko and Frances Thomson-Salo

A volume in the Psychoanalysis & Women Series for the Committee on Women and Psychoanalysis of the International Psychoanalytical Association

Routledge
Taylor & Francis Group
LONDON AND NEW YORK

First published 2017 by Karnac Books Ltd.

Published 2019 by Routledge
2 Park Square, Milton Park, Abingdon, Oxon OX14 4RN
52 Vanderbilt Avenue, New York, NY 10017

First issued in hardback 2019

Routledge is an imprint of the Taylor & Francis Group, an informa business

British Library Cataloguing in Publication Data

A C.I.P. for this book is available from the British Library

ISBN 13: 978-0-367-10418-4 (hbk)
ISBN 13: 978-1-78220-494-7 (pbk)

Edited, designed and produced by The Studio Publishing Services Ltd
www.publishingservicesuk.co.uk
email: studio@publishingservicesuk.co.uk

CONTENTS

PART III: SEXUAL DIVERSITY

ACKNOWLEDGEMENTS AND PERMISSIONS

We acknowledge the permission given by patients to use their material, either suitably de-identified or in composite vignettes.

We thank the publishers, Letra Viva, for permission to print an English translation of Alizade, M. (2010). "La liberación de la de la parentalidad en el Siglo XXI", in *Revista Imago Agenda, 140,* Buenos Aires; Teresa Rocha Leite Haudenschild, *Parentalidad y género en un caso de intersexualidad* (pp. 119–130); Teresa Lartigue, María Arrieta, and Teresa del Bosque and Dolores Montilla, *Parentalidad interrumpida. Un caso de muerte neonatal* (pp. 213–220), Ema Ponce de León Leiras, "Maternidad en la Adolescencia: perspectiva social y psicoanalítica" (2013) in *Cuadernos de Psiquiatría y Psicoterapia del Niño y del Adolescente, 56,* Madrid (pp. 67–76), and María Alejandra Rey, ?*Estamos embarazados? Fantasías desplegadas en el proceso de transferencia de embriones* (pp. 73–78).

We also thank the publishers of *Revista Brasileira de Psicanálise* for permission to include a translated version of Susana Muszkat's paper, "As neossexualidades e a discussao do modelo binario, *Revista Brasileira de Psicanálise, 48*: 106–114.

ABOUT THE EDITORS AND CONTRIBUTORS

Beatriz Agrest is a psychoanalyst and a full member of the Argentine Psychoanalytic Association (APA), and the International Psychoanalytical Association. She has presented papers, workshops, and panels about clinical work and theory on psychosomatics, adoption, and same-sex parenting at national and international conferences. She is the author of several articles published in the *Revista de Psicoanálisis* (APA), and others. She is a former member of the APA Research Group on Psychosomatics, and the Secretary of the Committee on Adoption, Same-sex Parenthood, and Sexual Diversity. She has been a member of the APA Publications Committee since 2013. She is a co-editor of *Homoparentalidades. Nuevas Familias* [Same-Sex Parenthood. New Families] (2010, 2nd edition, Lugar). Her books include the co-authored *El cuerpo en escena* (2012, Lumen), and *Parentalities*, co-edited with Eva Rotenberg (2014, Lugar).

Alcira Mariam Alizade (1943–2013) was a physician, psychiatrist, and full member and training analyst of the Argentine Psychoanalytic Association. From 1999–2001 she was the Latin American Co-Chair of the Committee on Women and Psychoanalysis (COWAP) and overall Chair of COWAP from 2001 to 2005. From 2006 to 2008 she was Scientific Secretary of FEPAL and published several books: *La sensualidad Femenina* (1992); *Clinica con la muerte* (1995); *Tiempo de Mujeres* (1996); *La Mujer Sola* (1998); *Lo Positivo en Psicoanálisis* (2002); *Adiós a la Sangre: Reflexiones Psicoanalíticas sobre la Menopausa* (2005); and *La pareja rota. Ensayo sobre el divorcio* (2010).

Patricia Alkolombre is a full member with Training Function of the Argentine Psychoanalytic Association (APA), liaison member for APA of the Committee on Women and Psychoanalysis (COWAP) of the International Psychoanalytical Association (IPA); Coordinator of the Eleventh COWAP Latin American Dialogue on "Parenthoods and Gender: Their influence on subjectivity", Buenos Aires, 2014. She is the editor and author of *Deseo de hijo. Pasión de hijo. Esterilidad y técnicas reproductivas a la luz del psicoanálisis* (Letra Viva, 2008), and *Travesías del cuerpo femenino. Un recorrido psicoanalítico en torno a temas de ginecología y obstetricia* (Letra Viva, 2011), which was officially declared "Of interest in the areas of culture and health" by the Legislature of the City of Buenos Aires and "Female sterility: her baby, her passion" *International Psychoanalytical Studies Organisation Journal*, 1997.

Guilherme Kirsten Barbisan, MD, graduated in medicine at Pontifical Catholic University and is a psychiatrist at the Hospital de Clínicas de Porto Alegre.

Emilce Dio Bleichmar, MD, PhD in the programme, "Principles and Developments in Psychoanalysis", is a member of the Argentine Psychoanalytical Association and the International Attachment Network. She is Head and Professor of Graduate Studies in Clinical and Psychoanalytical Psychotherapy of Child and Family and Head of the Women's Studies Department at ELIPSIS, Pontificia University, Madrid. Her publicatins include: *Fears and Phobias. Genesis Conditions on Infancy* (1982); *The Spontaneous Feminism of Hysteria* (1985); Award Essay, Woman Institute, Madrid. *Depression in Women* (1991); *Feminine Sexuality: From Child to Woman* (1998); *Manual of Psychotherapy of the Relation between Parent and Children* (2005); *Women Treating Women* (Ed.) (2011); "The place of motherhood in primary femininity" (in: *Motherhood in the Twenty-First Century* (2006)); "The psychoanalyst's implicit theories of gender" (in: *On Freud's Femininity* (2010)). She has also published numerous papers on femininity in Argentina, Brazil, the USA, Italy, and Spain.

Constanza Duhalde has a DEA (Master's degree) in Clinical Psychology, Paris V University, holds a Psychology PsD, University of Buenos Aires, and a Diploma in Infant Psychopathology, Paris XIII University. She is a professor and researcher at the University of Buenos Aires and a candidate in the Argentine Society of Psychoanalysis (SAP). She received the FEPAL award Psychoanalysis and Society (2008) for "Concebir, The Analytical Attitude To Face a Support Group of Infertile Couples. Meeting in the Community". She was a psychological adviser for Concebir (a support group of infertile patients) from 2001–2012. She is a member of the Argentine Center for Psychology and Reproduction. She is a co-author of *Así fue como llegaste*, children's books on medically assisted reproduction. She has written several papers on the psychological processes of parenthood, assisted reproduction, and the early parent–infant relationship, and has participated in national and international conferences.

Cláudio Laks Eizirik, MD, PhD, is a training and supervising psychoanalyst, Porto Alegre Psychoanalytic Society; Professor of Psychiatry, Medical School, Federal University of Rio Grande do Sul (UFRGS) and the MsC and PhD Program of Psychiatry and Behavioural Sciences, UFRGS); editor and author of the books *Key Papers on Countertransference* (Karnac, 2012); *O Ciclo da Vida Humana: uma perspective psicodinâmica* [The Human Life Cycle: A Psychodynamic Perspective] (Artmed, 2013); *Psicoterapia de Orientação Analítica-fundamentos teóricos e clínicos* [Analytically Orientated Psychotherapy: Theoretical and Clinical Bases)] (Artmed, 2015). He has also authored chapters, papers, research, and lectures on analytic training, analytic practice, psychoanalysis and culture, the process of ageing, psychoanalytic institutions, psychoanalysis, and gender. He is the former President of the IPA (2005–2009) and of FEPAL (1998–2000), the current Chair of the IPA Committee on Psychoanalysis and the Mental Health Field and received the Sigourney Award in 2011.

Leticia Glocer Fiorini has a Master's degree in Psychoanalysis (University of Salvador—APA) and is a training and supervising analyst of the Argentine Psychoanalytic Association and former president of this

Society. She was previously Chair of the Publications Committee of the IPA and the APA, and is the current adviser of the IPA Publications Committee. She was awarded the Celes Carcamo Prize in 1994. She is the author of: *Deconstructing the Feminine. Sexuality, Gender and Theories of Complexity* (2007), and *Lo femenino y el pensamiento complejo* [The Feminine and the Complex Thought] (2001). She co-edited *On Freud's "Femininity"* (2010); *The Experience of Time* (2009); *On Freud's "Mourning and Melancholia"* (2007), and was the General Editor of the *International Psychoanalysis Library* series and *Contemporary Freud. Turning Points and Critical Issues* series, published by the IPA Publications Committee (2005–2011). She has also published numerous papers in books and psychoanalytic journals on femininity, motherhood and sexual diversity in Spanish, English, Portuguese and Italian.

Teresa Rocha Leite Haudenschild is a training analyst and child and adolescent analyst of the Brazilian Psychoanalytical Society of São Paulo, and a full member of the International Psychoanalytical Association. She has worked in the field of clinical psychoanalysis for forty years, with particular focus on early symbolisation and the constitution of identity and psychosexuality. Her work on these topics has been published in Latin American and European journals. In 2015 she published the book *The First Gaze*, on the primary relationship, and in 2016 *Psychosexualities*, on femininity, masculinity and gender. She studied philosophy and worked as a journalist until she became interested in psychoanalysis. She is currently a representative of COWAP in the Brazilian Federation of Psychoanalysis.

Cândida Sé Holovko is a full member of IPA and the Brazilian Psychoanalytical Society of São Paulo (SBPSP); co-chair of COWAP for Latin America; a liaison member of COWAP-IPA with SBPSP, 2005–2008; Regional Editor for the Latin American journal *Calibán* (2012–2014); member in training with the Institute de Psychosomatique Pierre Marty de Paris; coordinator of a psychoanalytical psychosomatics group linked to the Institute of Paris; member of a psychosomatic study group at SBPSP; chief Editor of the Institute's Journal (*Jornal de Psicanálise*), 2009–2010, in which two volumes were dedicated to COWAP themes of Masculinities/Femininities (June and December, 2009). She has published on masculine and feminine psychosexuality, mind–body relations, and psychosomatics.

Silvia Jadur is a Psychology PsD, University of Córdoba, Argentina. She is a university professor in medicine and law. She is a founding member of Concebir (Support Group of Infertile Patients) 1996–2012, and received a FEPAL award for Psychoanalysis and Society (2008): "Concebir, The Analytical Attitude To Face a Support Group of Infertile Couples. Meeting in the Community", Award Siglo XXI Publishers. She wrote *Auxilio, el bebé no llega*! [Help, The Baby Does Not Arrive!]. She is a co-author of *Así fue como llegaste*, children's books on medically assisted reproduction. She was the Director of the Argentine Center for Psychology and Reproduction. Psychologist at Children's Hospital Dr. R. Gutierrez (1976–2000), and was the psychology chapter coordinator of the Argentine Society of Reproductive Medicine from 2012–2014. She has participated in national and international conferences.

Teresa Lartigue received her PhD in psychology at the Universidad Iberoamericana (Mexico), where she was Head of the School of Psychology (1977–1981). She is a training analyst and a child and adolescent psychoanalyst of the Mexican Psychoanalytic Association (APM), and a full member of the International Psychoanalytical Association (IPA). She is a former President of the APM (2002–2004); former Head of the Department of Reproductive Epidemiology at the National Institute of Perinatology, Mexico (2000–2007); a liaison member for COWAP, a former Director of the Mexican Institute of Psychoanalysis (2004–2006); a member of the Sub-Committee for the Evaluation of Research Proposals of the IPA and member of the sub-committee for Training in Research Methodology; a reviewer for Latin America of *The International Journal of Psychoanalysis*; an IPA College Research Fellow, and editor of the *Cuadernos de Psicoanálisis* journal of the APM.

Ema Ponce de León Leiras, PhD, is a clinical psychologist and a child, adolescent, and adult psychoanalyst. She is full member and training analyst of the Uruguayan Psychoanalytical Association and a member of the International Psychoanalytical Association. She represents Uruguay as a liaison member for the Committee on Women and Psychoanalysis. She lives in Montevideo and is the founder (in 1991) and director of "Clínica del Niño—Centro del Adolescente", an interdisciplinary clinic for the assistance of children and adolescents. She has been researching interdisciplinary interventions for children with difficulties in symbolising and severe developmental disorders. She works with infants and parents, couples, and adolescent mothers, has published many articles, and gives courses, lectures, and conferences in Europe and South America.

Susana Muszkat is a psychoanalyst, member of the Brazilian Society of Psychoanalysis of São Paulo; a member of the International Psychoanalytical Association (IPA); former co-chair of FEPAL (Latin American Psychoanalytic Federation) on Family and Couples Work Group (2010–2012); a current member of the IPA Family and Couples committee; a member of the Link Theory study and clinical work group on Families and Couples of the São Paulo Psychoanalytic Society; former review editor of the Brazilian Journal of Psychoanalysis (2007–2015); author of *Violence and Masculinity* (2011), and co-author of other books on family conflicts and violence and a number of articles in specialised journals.

María Alejandra Rey graduated in psychology from the Universidad de Buenos Aires and is an affiliated member of the Sociedad Argentina de Psicoanálisis (SAP, Argentine Psychoanalytical Society). She is the Assistant Director of the Media Committee of FEPAL and a Member of the Membership Communication Service Committee. She was IPA Media Coordinator of SAP 2009–2013, a member of the Scientific Committee of FEPAL 2012, of the local FEPAL Committee 2014 (Media Committee), a liaison member for the Committee on Women and Psychoanalysis, and a member of the Reading and Editing Committee of the Journal of the Argentine Psychoanalytical Society.

Ana Maria Rocca Rivarola graduated as a clinical psychologist from the University of Belgrano, Buenos Aires, Argentina. She is a full member and professor at the Institute of the Brazilian Psychoanalytic Society of São Paulo (SBPSP) and a Full Member of the International Psychoanalytical Association. Ana is also a Child and Adolescent Psychoanalyst for SBPSP and IPA and active in the COWAP community. She maintains a private practice of psychoanalysis for adults, adolescents, and children in addition to working with infant–parent interventions. She has published several articles and has presented papers at international conferences in Europe, USA, and South America. Currently, she lives in Campinas, São Paulo, Brazil.

Eva Rotenberg is a clinical psychologist and psychoanalyst, a full member of the Psychoanalytic Association (APA), and of the International Psychoanalytical Association, a child and adolescent psychoanalyst, and a liaison member for the Committee on Women and Psychoanalysis. She was chair of the Group on Parenthoods, FEPAL, 2014, and chair of the committee on psychoanalysis of children and adolescents, Chile, 2014–2015. She has been chair of the Committee on Adoption, Same-sex Parenthood, and Sexual Diversity at the Argentine Psychoanalytic Association from 2000. She is a former professor of the Masters in Psychoanalysis at the J. F. Kennedy University, Buenos Aires, and a visiting professor at foreign universities. She is the author of several articles published in the *Journal of Psychoanalysis* of the APA, Vertex, and the *Journal of Psychiatry*, author of many books, and co-author and co-editor of *Same-Sex Parenthoods, New Families* (Lugar, 2005). Her paper, "Organ transplant in children and adolescents" received honourable mention for scientific excellence at FEPAL.

Graciela Cardó Soria has a Master's degree in Theoretical Psychoanalytic Studies and is a psychoanalyst, a member of the Peru Psychoanalytic Society, and a liaison Member of COWAP. She teaches at the Centro de Psicoterapia Psicoanalítica de Lima CPPL and is a faculty member of PUCP.

Stefania Pigatto Teche, MD, MSc, has a Master's degree in Psychiatry from the Universidade Federal do Rio Grande do Sul (UFRGS) and specialised in analytical psychotherapy at the UFRGS. Currently, she works as a psychiatrist and psychotherapist at the Hospital de Clínicas de Porto Alegre.

Juan-Eduardo Tesone is a physician, psychiatrist, a full member of the Argentine Psychoanalytic Association and of the Société Psychanalytique de Paris; he teaches on the DUEFO of the Faculté de Médicine de la Pitié-Salpetrière, Paris VI, is an Associate Professor of the LASI School of Psychology of the University of Paris-Ouest Nanterre; a professor on the Masters and Doctoral courses, "The Disruptive and

Psychoanalysis", Salvador University, Buenos Aires; a professor on the Masters course, "Interdisciplinary Studies on Subjectivity" at the School of Philosophy and Letters, University of Buenos Aires, and a professor on the Postgraduate course, "Forensic Psychology", University of Economic and Social Sciences, Buenos Aires.

Frances Thomson-Salo, Associate Professor, trained in the UK as an adult and child psychoanalyst and is a member of the British Psychoanalytical Society and of the Australian Psychoanalytical Society, of which she is a past president. She is a training analyst, and was overall chair of the Committee on Women and Psychoanalysis for the International Psychoanalytical Association from 2009–2015. She is Series Editor for Karnac's "Psychoanalysis and Women" series and a member of the Editorial Board of the *International Journal of Psychoanalysis*.

Viviana Wainstein has a PsD in Psychology from Belgrano University, Buenos Aires, and a Master's degree in Sexology, Favaloro University, Buenos Aires. She is a professor at Belgrano University, Buenos Aires and a specialist in human reproduction, SAMER (Argentine Society of Reproductive Medicine). She received the FEPAL award Psychoanalysis and Society (2008): Concebir, the analytical attitude to face a support group of infertile couples. Meeting in the community. Award Siglo XXI Publishers. "Auxilio, el bebé no llega" (Help, the baby does not arrive!). She has contributed to a collection of popular science books. She was the psychological adviser of Concebir (a support group for infertile patients), 2004–2012. She is a member of CAPSIR (Argentine Center for Psychology and Reproduction), has written several papers on sexology, reproductive medicine, and psychoanalysis, and participated in national and international conferences.

SERIES EDITOR'S FOREWORD

Frances Thomson-Salo

I am pleased, as the former overall chair of the International Psychoanalytical Association's Committee on Women and Psychoanalysis (COWAP), for this book to be included in the growing library of the Karnac series "Psychoanalysis and Women", which presents revisions to current understandings. Otto Kernberg, when he was President of the IPA, set up COWAP in 1998 to explore scientific and political issues about the differences between women and men, with Joan Raphael-Leff as the foundational overall chair. A hallmark of COWAP is always being interested in engaging with other organisations and ideas, and opening up a reciprocal discussion. This book also extends the legacy of Mariam Alizade, who did so much to build up COWAP and the resulting output of books.

This book is based on the COWAP Latin American XI Dialogue on "Parenthoods and gender. Their influence on subjectivity", Buenos Aires, 2014. We thank the individual authors who have contributed so generously to this book, representing a range of work by a number of psychoanalysts from Latin America (FEPAL); they have furthered the debate in a way that will be felt to be respectful.

The chapters in this book offer a depth, breadth, and vibrancy of creative and scientific interest. The writing is often poignantly evocative and powerful, and, as psychoanalytic thinking and work become more complex, our understanding of the analytic process is deepened, with a greater awareness of broader ways of understanding the field. Much creativity has emerged from what has been studied, which we hope, in turn, will lead to a new therapeutic synthesis.

Last, we thank the International Psychoanalytical Association for their ongoing commitment to the work of the Committee on Women and Psychoanalysis.

Introduction

Cândida Sé Holovko and Frances Thomson-Salo

With the inauguration of psychoanalytic writing, Freud bequeathed a priceless heritage that each publication aims to expand, enlarge, and question. The Bionian expression, "public-action" (separated by a hyphen, the word has its meaning of a public and wide ranging action) comprises not only the moment of the interpretative process, when a mental phenomenon becomes a shared action, but equally so an important commitment involving any psychoanalyst with his or her analytic group. We now undertake the challenge—with joy and enthusiasm—to present to English-speaking readers a judicious and innovative work of renowned authors in Latin America. They have contributed to expand clinical–theoretical reflection in the field of psychoanalysis and to try to surmount the language barrier that has previously prevented access for a larger number of readers.

We have currently several theoretical models in psychoanalysis and bringing these models into a creative dialogue can be a way of not staying adrift. The sexual revolution of the 1960s, with the increased release of expressions of sexuality, combined with women's emancipation reinforced by the advent of contraceptives, have definitively separated sexuality from reproduction, and later, in the 1980s, the emergence of new reproductive technologies contributed to the emergence of new ways of forming families. All these changes observed in the contemporary society challenge long-established concepts in psychoanalysis, such as the Oedipus complex, parental functions, male and female psychosexuality, primal scene, affiliation, and so on. Roudinesco (2003), in her book, *A familia em desordem*, points out the evolution that the family institution has achieved over the years: from the patriarchal family with marriages of convenience for the maintenance and development of the family patrimony, followed by the modern family, inspired by marriage as a romantic liaison and a way of ensuring the love–sex relationship and the parents' responsibility in the education of the children, up to postmodern families from the 1960s onwards after the sexual revolution. In these families, based on finding sexual and emotional exchanges independent of the gender of its members, we find homoerotic couples who adopt children or who create them through assisted fertilisation; we also find single parent families, blended families, and so on. These postmodern families, in the words of Roudinesco, are the ones that most specifically have aroused controversy in the psychoanalytic or wider socio-cultural milieu.

For several years now, Latin American psychoanalysts have been discussing and writing about the urgency of revising theoretical and clinical concepts in the light of these new scenarios. In this sense we can say that the chapters of this book cover a wide range of concepts that show the uncertainty of contemporary clinical work. They revisit notions of parental functions that can broaden perspectives; they describe the neo-sexualities that require an innovative approach; they present the psychic consequences found in studies of and experiences with patients who make use of the technology of assisted fertilisation.

The longer first section of the book revisits psychoanalytic theories in the light of current thinking and societal developments in the area of sexuality and gender.

Leticia Glocer Fiorini, in the first chapter, proposes a rethinking of the Oedipus complex, a central concept to psychoanalysis, from the deconstruction of the concept of paternal function reviewing this function in contemporary families. Starting from the idea that the construction of sexual subjectivity is directly linked to the symbolic function, Glocer Fiorini aims to establish the difference between paternal function and "third party function". This is a terminology that she considers more accurate and comprehensive to avoid any relation with parental figures or real and imaginary substitutes that better describe symbolic operations. She decentralises the logic of binary thinking supported by power relationships (male–female, father–mother . . .) towards a vision that includes increasing heterogeneity and the logic of complexity, as its notion of plural and multicentric motherhoods. Glocer Fiorini shows, from a careful examination and innovative approach, the cultural–historical influences that have marked the conceptualisation of the paternal function and the need to recognise the symbolic subjectivity of the subjects that contribute to the emergence of the psyche within family ties, regardless of the gender of its participants. That a mother may exercise a third-party function can be seen in much infant–parent psychotherapy and infant research, matched by a desire for a child, is in line with Glocer Fiorini's suggestion that we need to work on where psychoanalysis abuts other disciplines.

Juan-Eduardo Tesone, in a thought-provoking chapter, "When a symbolic lack of parental functions produces pain without a subject", plunges us into the field of the not represented but psychically inscribed. With literary metaphors and clinical vignettes of cases of incest, he reveals the possibility of having psychic marks without a subject and gives us clues in this universe of the unremembered but marked. He states that, in traumatic situations, non-figuration is a defence against an unspeakable pain which is fixed and unable to be integrated and included in the network of representational associations. He proposes that the clinical work of the psychoanalyst is half way to a "conjectural science and a poiesis in which the subject appears increasingly . . .". In an original way, he explains how the production of dreams can function as memories of traumatic situations.

Emilce Dio Bleichmar, in her chapter examines aspects of the subjective world of mothers towards their children from theoretical and clinical psychoanalytic links and longitudinal studies of the dyadic mother-child relationship during the first five years. She observes patterns of early mother/baby interaction, and asks whether women are "prone to developing a severe superego when they become mothers". In an original approach she reveals her finding of increased persecutory anxiety in mothers' relationship with their babies in contemporary clinical work. About motherhood she says: "Motherhood becomes one of the early cores of the female ego ideal and one of the contents and objectives of her narcissistic system, providing self-esteem and efficacy to her representation of being female". She believes that the increase of information and demands of cultural ideas about maternal functions have generated more fantasies of the "bad internal mother" as opposed to the ideal mother who is always praised. Dio Bleichmar emphasises that the unconscious fantasy of being a bad mother predisposes mothers to develop more severe and primitive forms of superego, creating psychic defences to maintain the ideal of a good mother which ends up hurting and affecting the capacity for reflection in intersubjective exchanges with their babies, thus creating a vicious cycle.

Cândida Sé Holovko, in her chapter, "Secrets and revelations: vicissitudes of the maternal function", revisits the notion of "maternal function" proposed by the psychosomatic school of Paris, emphasising its usefulness in addressing the object introjection distortions with maternal function and of the transgenerational transmissions often found in eating disorders. From clinical vignettes of a young analysand with serious bulimic symptoms, she shows the transformation of compulsive bulimic acting towards a communication enriched by the expanded symbolic universe.

Teresa Lartigue, drawing on her long experience of care of, and research with, bereaved families after neonatal death emphasises, in her chapter, "Bereaved families after neonatal death", the importance of work with the countertransference in these situations of unspeakable pain from traumatic loss. In the moving and sensitive approach of a psychotherapeutic process offered over several years and with several interruptions to a young woman who lost her daughter soon after delivery, Lartigue shows in detail the vicissitudes of this particular analysis and what can be expected in similar situations: pain that can persist for many years; a reduction in the capacity for mentalisation; attacks to the immune system; difficulties in regulating affection; severe superego inducing self-punishment, and difficulties in interpersonal relations jeopardising the family structure. She emphasises the need for psychotherapeutic treatment for at least three years to enable the working through of the situations described.

Ema Ponce de León Leiras, in her chapter, "Adolescent maternity in a critical social context: a perspective from the psychoanalyst's *hilflosigkeit*", enables us to engage in psychoanalytic listening to adolescents in a context of total social, economic, and psychic privation, so that we reflect on the establishment of new clinical work. She emphasises that motherhood and adolescence, while having a unique subjective dimension, are also simultaneously social constructs. In a touching description of an analytic experience in a non-government organisation in Uruguay for teenage parents, Ponce de Léon Leiras wonders whether the search for pregnancy in a case she describes could be a way of making sexual aspects of life predominate over violence and death, promoting pulsional fusion of the erotic with Thanatos, the latter so prevalent in marginalised social sectors. Ponce de Léon Leiras affirms that every motherhood situation must be considered unique and it cannot be predicted that teenage motherhood will have negative consequences; on the contrary in many situations like this, motherhood is seen as an opportunity for social integration through a culturally valued role as a search for a certain kind of narcissistic balance. Ponce de Léon Leiras touches on the challenges psychoanalysts face in the twenty-first century: the opportunity to create clinical interventions favouring a real psychoanalytic interface with the demands of social reality in an exceptionally fruitful encounter.

We then move to the next section, which discusses some of the new family configurations that are seen worldwide. Patricia Alkolombre, building on clinical observations that have been researched for several years, develops innovative ideas about the place and the vicissitudes of the desire to have a child in men and women in relation to new parenthoods. Affected by the sacrificial aspect observed in several psychotherapies with people seeking assisted fertilisation, Alkolombre discusses the idea of having a child at any cost in an obsessive manner. Thus, she highlights the notion of the excess of pulsionality linked to reproductive functions and proposes the term "passion for children" as opposed to the desire for a child. To the extent that sex life is divorced from procreation, Alkolombre reminds us that different affiliation projects share the context of sexual diversity and she loosens the symbolic references that govern the identification of subjects. She discusses the introduction of the third, technical–medical element in this context of fertilisation and how it radically changes births and the impact of this on subjectivities.

On the same issue of assisted fertilisation treatments, Silvia Jadur and her colleagues—also with extensive experience in this matter—discuss in their chapter, "The role of 'donor' in assisted fertilisation treatments", the inevitable grief of the lost genetic illusion that the effect on subjectivity presses towards a libidinal reorganisation for reinvestment not only in the body image, but also of the psyche in the acceptance of a foreign gamete, both in women and men. They state that "the ghosts of the oedipal drama act out the castration anxieties in the face of the reality of the failed procreative function". They propose replacing the term "donor" by "contributor" for those men and women who supply the necessary reproductive cells. They indicate some effects of donor anonymity and their place in the medical discourse and subjectivity of individuals. They present some considerations about the desire to be a father and fantasies about infertility in men. Supported by research with families who used these techniques, they do not find differences between families conceived with gamete donors and families who have children as a result of natural conception.

Eva Rotenberg and Beatriz Agrest, in their chapter, "Parenthood for same-sex couples and gender definition in children", consider that the notion of parental function allows us to question the myth that the heterosexuality of the parents permits identification of children with their own biological sex or mental health. They believe that, in same-sex couples, one member can exercise the function of the third while the other would take care of the nurturing function—and both functions can be shared or even exchanged. They propose the term "parental true self" to refer to the function that allows the child to integrate the soma–psyche experience and subjectivation. The authors postulate that it is necessary to review the concept of affiliation owing to the enormous changes in consanguineous relationships and that it is affection that rules the desire to conceive or adopt children in same-sex couples. They emphasise the importance of the analyst's ethics and of science in these single-sex parenthood contexts and that there is not one single position on this subject in psychoanalysis. Different theories coexist which give different values to the anatomical sex differences and express different views of the Oedipus complex that should be reviewed in the light of contemporary practice.

Maria Alejandra Rey, in her chapter, "Are we pregnant? Fantasies displayed in the embryo transfer process", emphasises how technology has transformed relationships: egg and semen can be bought, embryos frozen, biological parents chosen, sex changed, bellies rented, a gay friend can donate semen to a lesbian couple, and so on, and she wonders how we perceive ourselves as parents in the present context. She considers that parental roles are continuously built and do not necessarily depend on the differences of sex, and that there is a difference drawn between parent and gamete donor according to the place they occupy in the child's mind. She refers to the emotional effects and fantasies in the cryopreservation of embryos and their transfer. She also believes that the new families are operating in an area without the myths and traditions of past generations, which implies both freedom and uncertainty.

In the third section, on sexual diversity, Teresa Rocha Leite Haudenschild, in her chapter, "Two in one: parenthood and gender in a case of intersexuality", reports a psychoanalytic process of intersexuality, of which there has been little discussion in the psychoanalytic literature. Her patient opted for the female sex while maintaining her physical bisexuality. Haudenschild discusses the creation and importance of primary and secondary bisexuality in the vicissitudes of gender designation. She believes that psychological criteria, such as the early relationship between unconscious and parental desires predominate over physical criteria in the future sexual orientation of these individuals. She emphasises that the parents' secondary psychical bisexuality and the extent to which they accept their child will determine the sexuality of those who are born with the anatomical characteristics of both sexes. In the analysis of the material presented, she suggests that the clinical work should focus on listening to the subject's uniqueness and, through the transference and countertransference processing, enable the emergence of anxieties and fantasies linked to the body.

Ana Rivarola, in her chapter, "The neuter gender and the setting up of psychosexuality", using the concept that Green (1983) formulated of the fantasy of neuter gender, presents rich clinical material where it is possible to see the psychoanalytic process of a patient with sexual undifferentiation who, as a result of the analysis, was able to reflect on her neutral position and feeling undifferentiated and, thus, have access to her own sexuality. This chapter revisits a very useful concept to be further explored when faced with unusual presentations that sexuality shows today, with some young people self-describing as asexual.

Cláudio Laks Eizirik, Stefania Pigatto Teche, and Guilherme Kristen Barbisan discuss "Countertransference in the psychodynamic psychotherapy of gender identity disorder patients". Here, we find the concept of countertransference in the psychoanalytic literature clearly reviewed, along with an exploration of its key role in analytic psychotherapy with, and evaluation for, sex reassignment surgery in transsexual individuals. Clinical illustrations present relevant topics for the treatment of gender dysphoria patients and show particular characteristics in projective identification and the introjective network established between psychotherapists, patients, and psychoanalyst supervisors. Eizirik and his colleagues point out the challenges faced by the psychotherapists of transsexuals, showing that the analytic field is created differently depending on their theories about female and male psychosexuality and the sex of the analyst and the patient's gender, which can lead to serious countertransference problems.

Susana Muszkat, in a surprising and unusual dialogue in her chapter, "Neo-sexualities and binary model debate", ushers in her writing by facing us with challenges of parental functions within the universe of same-sex parenting. Muszkat discusses socio-cultural and intrapsychic stereotypes that affect these relationships and invites analysts to reflect on what we now think of as father and mother and to think "outside the box while firmly anchored both in the analytic method and in the conception of an expanded psyche". The author understands neo-sexualities as modes of expressions of subjectivity, modes of expression that satisfy the subject-of-desire in aspects which are authentic and unique to each person, and these are not necessarily restricted to the binary heterosexuality system which she questions extensively in her chapter.

In the final section, we pay tribute to Mariam Alizade, Latin American co-chair of the Committee on Women and Psychoanalysis (1998–2001) and overall chair of COWAP from 2001–2005. An extraordinary human being and psychoanalyst, she contributed enormously not only with her writings and great enthusiasm for raising questions in our community, but also inspired psychoanalysts in both Latin America and in other regions of the world. Paying tribute to Alizade, Graciela Cardó Soria from the Sociedad Peruana of Psychoanalysis presents a biographical sketch of Alizade's life and work, emphasising her greatest theoretical contributions and mentioning those who influenced her work and personal development. In the passionate writing of a person who learnt a lot from her mentor, Graciela Cardó Soria describes the three central themes in Alizade's work: femininity (feminine sensuality), death (clinical work with the dying), and psychoanalysis and positivity.

Here, we republish Alizade's (2010) text, "The liberation of parentality in the twenty-first century", in which is listed many of the concerns related to the central theme of this book:

> These expressions of desire to generate a family organisation outside the social and cultural framework established centuries ago constitutes a movement of liberation. I propose to call for the liberation of parentality and for these phenomena to be included in new ways of parentality.

With her concept of the fourth complementary series Alizade (2005) stimulated the investigation of the social, cultural, political, factors present in the organisation of the human psyche. Writing about wisdom, Alizade said,

> The relativity of the universe and the limited uptake of science and the human faculties are able to generate in the human who tries to think the unthinkable, a dizziness, a wobble, a sudden loss of balance. It is perhaps the only way to achieve an instant and fleeting encounter with the infinite and the unthinkable. (p. 226, translated for this edition)

In this stimulating book, the reader will find some answers and considerable opening up of the ideas presented by our Latin American colleagues, who creatively cover familiar territories of our intimate concerns in psychoanalytic work in the contemporary world, and other areas that so far have been hardly explored. Here, the emphasis has been more on evolving parenthood and we need to hear what the children of such families tell us in their voice. Some readers might find that some "answers" are different from what might be expected, translated from a different tongue (see Tesone, Chapter Two) and we have tried to assist in a translation. (As one example, from the phrase "homoparentalities", more familiar to the Latin American and French analysts to the less elegant "single-sex parenthoods", in the interests of making these ideas more accessible.)

We wish you all good reading!

References

Alizade, A. M. (2005). *Adiós a la sangre: reflexiones psicoanalíticas sobre la menopausia*. Buenos Aires: Lumen.

Alizade, A. M. (2010). La liberación de la parentalidad en el Siglo XXI. In: *Neoparentalidades Revista Imago-Agenda*, n.140/junio, Buenos Aires.

Green, A. (1983). Le gendre neutre. In: *Narcissisme de vie, narcissisme de mort* (pp. 231–245). Paris: Éditions de Minuit.
Roudinesco, E. (2003). *A família em desordem* [The family in disorder]. Rio de Janeiro: Jorge Zahar.

PART I

REVISITING PARENTAL FUNCTIONS

CHAPTER ONE

The decline of the father: paternal function or third-party function?*

Leticia Glocer Fiorini

Introduction

Recent decades have seen much discussion regarding the anthropological, social, cultural, and psychological meaning of the nuclear family and its functions. Some of the themes explored clearly concern the psychoanalytic field, especially if we consider that the Oedipus complex replicates the organisation of the nuclear family. More specifically, in reference to the functions of its members, mother and father, both practical, everyday functions as well as those exercised on a symbolic level. These two levels are different, but there is a correlation between them.

Although these debates date quite far back, they have been intensified by diverse and very significant factors that we observe in contemporary societies, mainly occidental, but presently expanding to other cultures. Some changes in family organisation (single-sex parents, assembled and single parent families) are widely known, to which we may add the frequent phenomena of "castling" in everyday

* A version of this chapter was published as "Deconstructing the concept of paternal function" [translated for this edition] in *Revista de Psicoanálisis LXX*, 4: 671–681, 2013. This chapter also appears as "Deconstructing the paternal function—paternal function or third-party function?" in Glocer Fiorini, L. (2017). *Sexual Difference in Debate: Bodies, Desires and Fictions*. London: Karnac.

functions of mothers and fathers, since work and caring for children are not tasks assignable to fathers and mothers, respectively. Also quite significant are changes in the place occupied by women, again mainly in occidental societies, from women's access to the workforce, marked by the First World War, to the use of contraceptives. We might add the advances in techniques of assisted fertilisation that allow not only heterosexual couples, but also homosexual and non-conventional couples, as well as single persons, to have biological children. Changes in legislation in many countries also induce us to reflect on the influence of this topic on our practice.

Filial and kinship orders are involved, as well as the different meanings of the mechanisms of inheritance. We are also led to rethink the concepts of the centrality of the phallus and of sexual difference as a key, in some theoretical views, to access to a symbolic universe. In this line, we include the need to rethink the Oedipus complex in an expanded and trans-familial way (Glocer Fiorini, 2007, 2010a,b, 2015).

Although the relation between these changes and psychoanalysis is not direct, since psychoanalysis has its own central lines inherent to the discipline, neither is it pertinent to consider them separate fields without mutual influence. We believe that a complex relation exists between the psychoanalytic field and other disciplines on which we need to work. This is an interdisciplinary issue.

In this frame, many questions arise which are the starting point of our proposal:

1. In view of new modalities of family organisation, new and not so new sexual and gender diversities, changes in the place of women and, therefore, also of men in occidental societies (fragmentary changes, it is true, but changes advancing as a tendency), how do we reflect on the issue of the so-called decline of the father in contemporary societies?
2. Is this a decline or is it that new ways to exercise a symbolic function are germinating? In other words: are paternal function and symbolic function parts of an inseparable equation?
3. Can this symbolic function be exercised by others and, if so, may we legitimately call it a "paternal" function, even in the symbolic sense attributed to it?
4. Are there echoes of patriarchal societies in the conceptualisation of this function? This implies the need to consider whether psychoanalysis is outside the episteme of our time or whether, to the contrary, it is marked by it, as occurs in the case of other disciplines.

5. Is the paternal function structural in character, its variations being manifestations of our era? Or, alternatively, is it the symbolic function itself that is structural in character?

These questions may be added to other questions that also affect daily work in our consulting rooms. Is it the same to have two mothers or two fathers? Is a single parent family the same as a nuclear family? How does the parents' gender influence functions called paternal and maternal? Furthermore, what is the involvement of the sexuated body?

In the perspective that the construction of sexuated subjectivity in a symbolic sense is involved, I propose (Glocer Fiorini, 2013) to call the "paternal" function the third-party function in order to avoid any equation with a real and imaginary figure of parents or substitutes and because the terms paternal function, paternal metaphor or Name (Names) of the Father (Lacan, 1970, 2005) have ideological echoes and implications that heavily affect the process of the cure.

This does not mean that we ignore the effects of the lack of father in clinical work, but it does mean clarifying the interpretative and ideological quantum by which a symbolic operatory becomes a structural universal.

In papers on this subject, paternal function is not discriminated from symbolic function because they are intimately welded together and made equal. Our position is that "paternal" function is *one* of the forms, but not the only one, taken by the symbolic function or functions indispensable for the construction of subjectivity.

Therefore, the central hypothesis and objective of this paper is to establish the difference between paternal function and third-party function. Although they both refer to a symbolic operatory, the former is indissolubly linked to the "name of the father" and, more concretely, to the father or father substitutes. However, a problem still persists: why cling to the term "paternal" to describe an eminently symbolic function?

A change of paradigm

We base our proposal on work to deconstruct the so-called paternal function. We have joined this objective with the aim of studying its genealogy, in the direction of analysing determinations that have converged on what is now called the paternal function.

As I pointed out, interest in this topic was generated by changes observed in current societies, in certain cultures and sub-cultures, concerning the emergence of new family configurations and the large visibility of so-called sexual and gender diversities in contemporary societies. The way those functions are exercised is a crucial issue, since it involves thinking about whether some subjects might or might not be excluded from the symbolic universe, depending on the way we think about these functions. This is a challenge for our clinical work. We also need to review the paternal function in the nuclear family of contemporary societies.

In this context, it is indispensable to consider whether we are looking at a change of paradigm. We do not take this term in the strict sense proposed by Kuhn (1971), which later generated different debates. We do, however, focus on one aspect of his proposal that we consider fundamental. In view of historical changes in human relations, some of which I have already mentioned, we find changes in models of thinking and in the types of logic that support them: from monocausal deterministic logic to multi-determinations; from multi-determinations to logics of heterogeneities and of intersections (of the "in between"). In our opinion, this points to a change of paradigm for understanding the place and functions of fathers and mothers without forcing theory. It also involves decentring binary thought that localises certain functions in fathers and mothers, and advancing towards thinking in complexity (Glocer Fiorini, 1994, 1998, 2007; Morin, 1990).

Concerning the concept of structure, I do not refer to structuralism in the sense of proposing eternal and ahistorical structures to explain the pregnancy of the paternal function. On the contrary, I support the proposal of Sartre (1991), who considers structure as mediation. Sartre considers structures as false syntheses and structural proposals as a moment in an anthropology that should be simultaneously historical and structural.

The decline of the paternal function

As we have said, an idea is circulating forcefully: the decline of the paternal function. Clinical and social problems are attributed to this:

diverse pathologies, all types of violence, wars. This figure that has been in crisis since the beginnings of modernity is now yielding, mainly in occidental societies, to other organisations of the practice of parenting.

The first question is: was it lost or did it perhaps never exist with the effectiveness that is assumed or in the way it is imagined? If it did exist, as we view it in the history of humanity from antiquity to the present, we might say that this pregnancy of the father has not been able to avoid socio-political crises, events of extreme violence, incest, abuse of power, or challenges to norms dictated by societies concerning sexual difference. From this perspective, we may speak of nostalgia for something we never had.

This demands genealogical analysis of the origin of the notion of paternal function and this is the aim of this chapter. I approach this analysis from two points of access: (1) from discourses and significant systems provided by the history of culture; (2) from the psychoanalytic viewpoint, and then I analyse possible relations between these two aspects.

First, the Bible teaches that Eve came from Adam's rib in the official version. We also recall that Aristotle considered that men were Form and women Formless; also that only as late as the Council of Trent did the Church recognise that women had a soul. Or that Spinoza wondered whether ethics could be attributed to women. We find innumerable examples in the history of culture in relation to a dichotomous and hierarchical division of the sexes, which leads us to consider how the figure of the capitalised Father came to be constructed, different from fathers in everyday experience. All considered, could the paternal function, even conceived in a symbolic register, rid itself of connotations derived from a patriarchal society whose characteristics have been thoroughly studied by different disciplines? Could it also divest itself of religious connotations linked to God the Father?

The psychoanalytic viewpoint

For these reasons and now turning to a discussion of the psychoanalytic viewpoint, we need to analyse the elements on which this concept is based in clinical work and psychoanalytic theory, its premises and blind spots. Freud devotes several works to the subject of the father: *Totem and Taboo* (1912–1913), *The Future of an Illusion* (1927c), and *Moses and Monotheism* (1939a), among others.

> It had laid open to view the father who had all along been hidden behind every divine figure as its nucleus. Fundamentally, this was a return to the historical beginnings of the idea of God. Now that God was a single person, man's relation to him could recover the intimacy and intensity of the child's relation to his father. (Freud, 1927c, p. 19)

He clearly points out its connection with religious sentiment and the need of most men and women to find support in these beliefs in their original helplessness and defencelessness. The protective god that may sometimes be vengeful and authoritarian is God the Father. In this sense, the paternal function is constituted as such in solidarity with patriarchal societies and religious sentiment. Also in this regard, it is a *construction.*

Totem and Taboo (Freud, 1912–1913) is one of the list of Freud's works that propose a mythical explanation, never proved by anthropologists or ethnologists, concerning the pregnancy of the father in androcentric societies. Belinsky (1997) considers that the originary father of the horde is created simultaneously with the enunciation of the myth. He points out that the Father was murdered because he had to be immortal rather than *vice versa.* He adds that Freud founds a myth situated in the perspective of patriarchal logic. In that context, this myth of the origins is an explanation of the patriarchal origin of society and culture rather than an explanation of their origin in general.

We need to remember that Freud never spoke of paternal function, although he did investigate the individual, cultural, and collective genealogy of the search for a father based on religious sentiment and founding father myths, also discussing the effects of the lack of a father, a category different from that of the capitalised Father. When he analyses *Leonardo Da Vinci and a Memory of His Childhood,* Freud (1910c) alludes to the lack of father in the origin of homosexuality, a lack of father that is different from terms such as the law of the Father (Lacan, 1970) with their patriarchal connotations.

Mitchell and Rose (1982) consider that Freud described the patriarchal system accurately and fairly. We would add that the paternal function is the heir of the *paterfamiliae* of Roman Law, based on the hierarchical division of the sexes involved in relations of power and domination.

At this point, we meet with another problem: the importance assigned in the psychoanalytic field to changes, already mentioned, occurring rapidly, mainly in occidental societies, in relation to the place of women, other family models different from the nuclear family, the rapid growth and spread of biotechnologies and their impact on contemporary maternities and paternities, as well as sexual and gender presentations that challenge the notion of sexual difference. In the latter case, would children of non-conventional couples or single parent families be excluded from the symbolic interweave?

Here, we have two options: either we consider these changes fashions of our era that do not alter the essence of psychoanalysis, or we wonder whether psychoanalysis might rethink some categories that are being challenged.

No doubt the concept of paternal function responds to many determinations. We could say that it originates in the need to explain the child's symbolic separation from the mother in the mother–father–child triangle. The concept of the symbolic father arises from it. However, there is another issue that is obscured, which is that the mother is placed in a lateralised position, situated structurally in a place belonging only to drives: the child's entrapment with no chance to generate a separation. Not only is this not observed universally in clinical practice, but it also disavows the possibility that a mother may possess sufficient symbolic reserves to allow her to desire and promote this separation as well (Benjamin, 1995).

These symbolic reserves do not refer, in my opinion, to the mother's ability to include the "paternal" function in her psyche, but, rather, to her ability to exercise a symbolic function *per se* and to support as her own the necessary symbolic third-party operatories to establish distinctions, differences, and separations in a symbolic sense. This indicates the complexity of the maternal position, which might be partly ensnared in drives but partly contains the potential to develop symbolic functions of separation from her child. For this reason, we proposed (Glocer Fiorini, 2001, 2007) the concept of plural and multi-centric maternities.

In regard to each individual boy or girl, we know that the real father might or might not fulfil these functions; in the same way, the mother might be fusionally adhered to her child or might desire to establish creative separations.

In our current legalities, it certainly creates less conflict when we think of the classic nuclear family and traditional interpretations: the devouring-drive mother and the separating, symbolic father. However, I believe that if we detach symbolic functions from terms that we can no longer apply legitimately, we may then be free to think about fathers, mothers, and their functions in a different way.

For all these reasons, we consider that the term third-party function describes more precisely these symbolic operatories.

The nature–culture debate

Returning to the specifically psychoanalytic sphere, the father, if thought of as exercising the paternal function (because he obviously might not fulfil it), accomplishes the objective of separating the child from the mother, of cutting off this relationship centred on thinking of the child as the mother's phallus, a relation that only the paternal metaphor could cut off. This permits the child's insertion into an exogamic symbolic universe. This is a concatenation of notions that apparently cannot be unlinked.

We also know that, since it is a function, it may be exercised by others who are not the father, either because of his absence or his deficiency. Therefore, it is a function that we call "paternal" but may be exercised by others. It may even be exercised by the mother. Consequently, as we pointed out, we might wonder why it is called "paternal" if it is a symbolic function.

The answer to this question requires further explanation since it presents a problem that we need to overt. It is emphasised that the mother may exercise it if she has internalised the father figure as a symbolic function. This obviously situates the mother in the place of Nature: a mother who retains her child and from whom only the intervention of Culture, the symbolic Father, is able to rescue the child, locked in a sort of deadly embrace. In other words, the condition that proposes that the introduction of the Father into the mother's mind implies that she accepts separation from the child is a patriarchal interpretation that again pushes the mother back into the place of pure Nature.

There is, however, another option, which I believe we need to contemplate: that the mother might exercise this symbolic function that may promote the separation of the child as a desire of her own. In other words, we need to recognise the mother as a subject. Functions do not belong exclusively to any gender, although there is predominance owing to different circumstances. This involves much more than the fact that the mother has internalised the "paternal" function. It involves recognising a symbolic function in the mother in her own right. This function does not belong to her, or to the father, even though she might be capable of exercising it. This assumes that although the child may be a phallus-child at some moments, she/he may also be a child in the sense of an other, at other moments. If the latter fails, there will certainly be problems, just as there would be if the paternal function failed because the father or substitute failed to recognise the child as an other. For all these reasons, when we speak of the symbolic father, we are also speaking of the mother and redefining her functions.

The notion of phallus-child responds to an essential lack in the mother that can only be compensated precisely by a phallus-child. This merits discussion. The attribution of a lack concerning women, which is no more than an interpretation, is equivalent to infantile sexual theories that are an interpretation of sexual difference. "Has or has not" is, in any case, a clinical fact that may appear in the course of an analysis. From this conception derives the concept of the phallic mother, ensnaring and devouring, who cannot give up the phallus-child. These infantile sexual theories may be preserved in the adult and also in the form of theoretical explanation in psychoanalysis. In relation to this issue, we took the concept of Deleuze (1995) concerning desire. This author considers that desire arises not from any essential lack but, conversely, lack is configured in relation to a desiring field.

We may say that dichotomous divisions such as nature–culture linked to mother–father, respectively, accentuate stereotypes of patriarchal societies: the phallic mother who clings to her child without letting the child go and the symbolic father who cuts them apart. When the nature–culture opposition is made an equivalent of mothers and fathers it is an obstacle to thinking about the construction of subjectivity. Tubert (1997) points out a radical asymmetry in occidental thought between maternal and paternal principles: the former is identified with nature whereas the latter is elevated to the category of a spiritual principle, as we observe in diverse domains such as philosophy, monotheistic theology, and linguistics.

This dichotomy responds to binary thought, which involves power relations (Glocer Fiorini, 1994, 2007). We have also shown (Glocer Fiorini, 2010c) that these binary polarities support the dichotomy between subject of desire *vs.* object of desire and subject of knowledge *vs.* object of knowledge, both made equivalent to masculine–feminine polarity. These are equivalences that we need to deconstruct.

It would be impossible to analyse this issue without referring to hierarchical and power relations between the sexes that impregnate the history of civilisation and construct signifiers and culture (Bourdieu, 2001). The figure of the father of the patriarchy, in charge of educating women and children and determining their fate, is constructed on the asymmetry of these relations.

Tort (2008) pointed out that psychoanalysis identifies the psychic device of "law", which ensures the institution of the subject, with the paternal function. He notes that "The Father" is the name of a historic solution that is being displaced. He proposes that when, on the contrary, we perceive that the paternal solution is not the only relation that subjects may have with law but is a totally particular moment, we might be able to engender an entirely different conception of subjectivity. He adds that it is indispensable for us to differentiate a psychoanalytic approach that opens theoretical and clinical perspectives from whatever constitutes subtle forms of normalisation.

Advancing further, is it necessary to rescue the child from a deadly embrace? Or could it be, as Héritier (2007) suggests, that what is at stake is patriarchal appropriation of the child?

Therefore, if there are sufficient symbolic, sublimatory, and creative resources in the mother, she may exercise this function, provided that she is positioned beyond an exclusively narcissistic field. This is too well known, but is always attributed to the introduction of the law in the mother by the Father. For this reason, preservation of the term "paternal" function is a way to universalise something that is actually a symbolic operatory indivisible from a certain type of society and ideology.

If this is true, and, as I pointed out, this is my proposal, paternal function should actually be called symbolic third-party function, independent of the person who exercises it and beyond impoverishing dichotomies. I consider that the concept of a third, symbolic function places it in a true category as a function that is autonomous in relation to the person exercising it. Otherwise, the risk is that we may essentialise something that is a historical construction. As Castoriadis (1984) proposed, there is interplay between "the instituted and the instituting" in social and cultural organisation. This refers to movement and changes that are essential for thinking about the "paternal function" in psychoanalysis.

For this reason, I believe that instead of speaking of new modalities of "paternal" function, which eternalises something that is contingent, we need to speak in terms of new modalities in the exercise of a symbolic function.

Finally, this does not imply the exclusion of fathers or functions they may fulfil. The search for a father marks many subjectivities. On the contrary, it involves an expansion of the role of fathers in both their symbolic and caring functions.

To conclude, since the way the paternal function is conceptualised has effects on analytic process, we have proposed to deconstruct the concept of paternal function and to dismantle its equation with symbolic function and law(s) that regulate a subject's insertion in a context of social ties. For this reason, we propose to call this function the third-party, symbolic function. It may assume different historic forms, one of which is the paternal function. Therefore, it needs a process of deconstruction in order to redefine terms and functions not only to include in it new forms of parenthood, but also to help us to review clinical *impasses* that might occur in classical forms of the nuclear family if we fail to make this necessary revision of certain psychoanalytic concepts in favour of new constructions.

References

Belinsky, J. (1997). Arquitectura de un mito moderno. In: S. Tubert (Ed.), *Figuras del Padre* (pp. 63–93). Barcelona: Cátedra.

Benjamin, J. (1995). *Like Subjects, Love Objects: Essays on Recognition and Sexual Difference*. New Haven, CT: Yale University Press.

Bourdieu, P. (2001). *Masculine Domination*. Cambridge: Polity.

Castoriadis, C. (1984). Psychoanalysis: project and elucidation. In: *Crossroads in the Labyrinth*. Brighton: Harvester.

Deleuze, G. (1995). *Conversaciones*. Valencia: Pre-textos.

Freud, S. (1910c). *Leonardo Da Vinci and a Memory of His Childhood. S. E., 11*: 59–138. London: Hogarth.

Freud, S. (1912–1913). *Totem and Taboo. S. E., 13*. London: Hogarth.

Freud, S. (1927c). *The Future of an Illusion. S. E., 21*: 3–56. London: Hogarth.

Freud, S. (1939a). *Moses and Monotheism. S. E., 23*: 3–137. London: Hogarth.

Glocer Fiorini, L. (1994). La posición femenina: una construcción heterogénea [The feminine position: a heterogeneous construction]. *Revista de Psicoanálisis, 51*: 587–603.

Glocer Fiorini, L. (1998). The feminine in psychoanalysis: a complex construction. *Journal of Clinical Psychoanalysis, 7*: 421–439.

Glocer Fiorini, L. (2001). El deseo de hijo: de la carencia a la producción deseante. *Revista de Psicoanálisis, LVIII*(4): 965–976.

Glocer Fiorini, L. (2007). *Deconstructing the Feminine. Psychoanalysis, Gender and Theories of Complexity*. London: Karnac.

Glocer Fiorini, L. (2010a). Sexualidades nómades y transgénero: un desafío a la polaridad masculino/femenino. In: B. Zelcer (Ed.), *Diversidad Sexual* (pp. 57–76). Buenos Aires: Lugar Editorial.

Glocer Fiorini, L. (2010b). Presentaciones cambiantes de la sexualidad. *Revista Uruguaya de Psicoanálisis, 111*: 44–53.

Glocer Fiorini, L. (2010c). The analyst's meta-theories concerning sexual difference and the feminine. In: L. Glocer Fiorini & G. Abelin-Sas Rose (Eds.), *On Freud's "Femininity"* (pp. 79–96). London: Karnac.

Glocer Fiorini, L. (2013). Deconstruyendo el concepto de función paterna. Un paradigma interpelado [Deconstructing the concept of paternal function]. *Revista de Psicoanálisis, LXX*(4): 671–682.

Glocer Fiorini, L. (2015). *La diferencia sexual en debate. Cuerpos, deseos y ficciones*. Buenos Aires: Lugar Editorial. [*Sexual Difference in Debate: Bodies, Desires and Fictions*. London: Karnac, 2017].

Héritier, F. (2007). *Masculino-Femenino II*. Buenos Aires: Fondo de Cultura Económica.

Kuhn, T. S. (1962/ 1971). *The Structure of Scientific Revolutions*. Chicago, IL: University of Chicago Press.

Lacan, J. (1970). *Las Formaciones del Inconsciente*. Buenos Aires: Nueva Visión.

Lacan, J. (2005). *De los Nombres del Padre*. Buenos Aires: Paidós.

Mitchell, J., & Rose, J. (1982). *Feminine Sexuality: Jacques Lacan and the École Freudienne*. New York: Norton.

Morin, E. (1990). *Introducción al Pensamiento Complejo*. Barcelona: Gedisa.

Sartre, J.-P. (1991). *Critique of Dialectical Reason. Vol. I*. London: Verso.

Tort, M. (2008). *Fin del Dogma Paterno*. Buenos Aires: Paidós.

Tubert, S. (1997). El nombre del padre. In: S. Tubert (Ed.), *Figuras del Padre* (pp. 31–61). Barcelona: Cátedra.

CHAPTER TWO

When a symbolic lack of parental functions produces pain without a subject

Juan-Eduardo Tesone

> "I suffer knowing I am involved in myself, and I suffer this in a suffocation of conclusions. . . . The only real art is that of construction"
>
> (Pessoa, 2002, translated for this edition)

The concept of fantasy in Freud inevitably refers to the concept of perception, based on what is inscribed in the subject from conscious or unconscious perceptions. Now, if Freud considers that in fantasy construction, as in dreams, the subject is always present, could we say that a person may have sensory experiences, events that remain outside the subjective field and, therefore, of fantasy? Furthermore, if this were true, what meta-psychological status and implications would they have in clinical work with whatever provokes a lasting psychic effect, an effect of memory outside the field of the lifting of repression and of fantasy? Is there parental lack that could produce psychic inscription without a subject (Tesone, 2009)?

Psychoanalysis in the past twenty years has turned its interest not only towards fantasy, but also to what may be figured or represented, in opposition not so much to what may not be represented as to what is not represented but, rather, inscribed. As highlighted by Sara and Cesar Botella (1992), non-representation originates neither in repression nor in denial and is not an effect of the castration complex or the product of an ego mechanism. It is by taking into consideration a hole, a negativity manifested in psychic dynamics in the form of an alteration of a process, most frequently expressed as a defect in thinking, that they postulate it as being like memory without memories. In this regard, we re-encounter Bion's (1962) proposals regarding thoughts without a thinker.

The field of the traumatic paradigmatically questions what cannot be represented, putting the classical analytic device of making conscious the unconscious in tension and revealing that in this clinical work it is not enough to lift repression in order to enable a somewhat anaemic trace to become memory. Traumatic experience sometimes generates emptiness of figuration that swallows up any possible form of representation, prior to fantasy. How does inscription acquire perception of the disruptive fact? My objective is to open a road rather than to indicate an itinerary with respect to this enquiry.

"Her childhood had injured her to such a degree that she could not evoke it", suggests Quignard (1998, p. 35, translated for this edition), referring to Némie, the protagonist of his novel, *Vie Secrète* [Secret Life]. I would add, perhaps because pain might sweep away the possibility to represent it, too; non-figuration is a defence against unspeakable pain. "What pain are you talking about if I didn't feel it . . ." could be the eloquent phrasing of this extreme psychic resource.

Duras (1964, p. 47) writes of Lol V. Stein in her novel, *Le Ravissement de Lol V. Stein*, "suffering had not found in her anywhere to slip out". Later in the same novel (p. 58, translated for this edition) she wonders, "But what does suffering without a subject mean?".

In his paper, "Fear of breakdown", Winnicott (1974) states that this is perhaps fear of a past event whose experience has not yet been undergone. The need to go through this experience is equivalent to what, in the analysis of neurotics, might be the need to remember.

As we know, experiences are traumatic when they are disruptive, as Benyakar (2006) suggests, having caused processes of binding to fail, rendering them incapable of representation. Outside of what may be figured or represented, traumatic experience escapes the domain of the symbolic and, therefore, remains suspended in a fixed, slowed down time that cannot be worked through. Benyakar (2006) states that the essence of the traumatic is invasion of the psyche by something heterogeneous, extraneous, impossible to metabolise, and which, thereby, transforms into something of one's own.

What is the status of something that has been experienced without being experienced, which is part of the psyche without being represented, that not having been symbolised has not been able to be subjectivised? In any case, we are far from fantasy and the intrinsic inclusion of the subject in the scene to which Freud referred.

Subjects who have suffered disruptive experience that has become traumatic are disquieting because they remain in a "no man's land" on the border, more unstructured than structured, yet not de-structured; they cannot decide to belong to any official classification, deprived of these letters of nobility. Or, rather, the agency of the letter is not written in a precise way.

We know that the concept of polyphony, elaborated by Bajtin, inspired by Mardi Gras literature and taken up by Ducrot in linguistics, questions the oneness of the speaking subject. Ducrot (1984) draws a distinction between the speaker, the being who produces an enunciate attributed to it, *vs.* the subject of the enunciation, which might make several voices speak. It is possible, Ducrot tells us, that some enunciations might not be the product of an individual subjectivity. In Ducrot's idea of enunciation, voices may appear that are not those of the speaker. These beings that might be expressed through an enunciation, even though no precise words may be attributed to them, Ducrot terms "enunciators". I ask, however, as a counterpart to polyphony, may enunciators exist without a speaker?

When Roussillon (1995) postulated the dual aspect of psychic reality, he tried to answer this question. On the one hand, the psyche concerns experiences that have successfully been inscribed in the representative system, subjected to the functioning of the pleasure–unpleasure principle and of the integration of wish fantasies made conflictual by consideration of reality; on the other hand, the psyche concerns what remains outside the integrative work of the life drives: split-off primary traumatic zones, crypts in search of representations which, being erratic, are subjected to the automatism of repetition. Meanwhile, deadly anxiety is expressed in pure form, as psychosomatic illness, or as repetition compulsion.

I disagree with Ferenczi (1984) when he states that trauma generates an arrest of all psychic activity. This total paralysis, he considers, includes the "arrest of perception and at the same time of thought". He adds that "it is not possible to defend against an impression that has not been received" and postulates that "no memory trace will remain of these impressions, not even in the unconscious, and consequently the origins of the commotion will be inaccessible to memory" (p. 551, translated for this edition).

I understand that Ferenczi is referring to difficulty in calling up remembrance memory. However, I do not think that there is no psychic inscription. Perhaps it is a question of what, in neuroscience, is called implicit memory, that is, sensations lacking representations or emotions that have never been memorised.

Freud (1937d, p. 260) stated that

> even things that seem completely forgotten are present somehow and somewhere, and have merely been buried and made inaccessible to the subject. Indeed, it may, as we know, be doubted whether any psychical structure can really be the victim of total destruction.

That is to say that he does not consider that no inscription has been produced. The outstanding question is in what way this occurs.

Moreno (2002, p. 43) states that "the subject is affected by what is not represented", and he calls this element an "indeterminate feature without representation". Thus, a feature, according to Moreno, is "pure difference without representation that becomes a mark when a fact gives it meaning". If a feature is to become a mark, he writes, a sanction must transform it into this mark, which separates the unmeaningful from the meaningful. I think that this difference consists in an affect suffered but, since it cannot be represented, it cannot be experienced and, thereby, be bound to a representation. It is as if the person had not been able to become aware of the trace of this feature, to such an extent that, in order to reveal the mark left in the psyche, this person must find a meaning to bind it.

The psychic apparatus tries to bind erratic anxiety, and representation is perhaps the most elaborate way to deactivate it. "In dreams we feel no horror that a sphinx is oppressing us, we dream of a sphinx in order to explain the horror we feel", writes Borges (1974b, p. 805, translated for this edition). The psychic apparatus does not permit anxiety to remain floating. Anxiety is Pirandellian, as in *Six Characters in Search of an Author* (Pirandello, 1993); anxiety is searching for a representation to which it can be referred as its author. It is for this reason that, in clinical work with traumatic experience, construction takes on the value of interpretation. That is to say that it is not necessarily a search for construction that possesses historical truth, but, rather, it plays a role in the dynamics of the psychic apparatus. Freud (1937d) even proposes that the term reconstruction should replace the term interpretation.

It is no longer a question of re-establishing by deduction the original form of the text as Freud underscored in *Totem and Taboo* (1912–1913) or in *Moses and Monotheism* (1939a). Something is missing in a much more radical way: the archaeological metaphor of finding layers unmodified and stratified but perfectly recognisable meets its limit (Press, 2008).

It is less a matter of giving interpretative value to the traumatic scene, the perceptive conformation of which is impossible to ascertain, than of listening to pain awaiting suffering that the subject might finally experience; then, the subject may take the floating enunciate and make it his or her own as an experienced enunciation.

Who is narrating?

In the words of several young girls who had suffered incest, followed up in a centre specialising in outpatient psychotherapy for this complex problem, which I was responsible for co-ordinating for several years, the traumatic appears (Tesone, 2005) as a filigree throughout the narration of excitement that had been generated in the girl's body by a burglary: physical stimulation breaking in from the outside without her consent or desire. This body, which responds in an uncontrolled way to external excitation, becomes itself an external body, through a diversification of the ego. This body that made her feel things is not her body. It is a body she does not recognise as her own. The excitement produced does not, however, make her desirous, since it is desubjectivising excitation. It is violence added to the violence of penetration. Desire is not involved; it is excitation stolen from her and a fraud as well, since it triggers drive excitation without the subject's consent. The height of trauma is this brutish and brutal encounter with a desymbolising event that does not allow the subject to ensure the continuity of living (Assoun, 1999). The body thereby acquires an extraterritorial quality with a jurisdiction of its own, which requires punishment. It is triply traumatic: due to the burglary and hypercathexis of the act in itself, due to alienating excitation produced without consent or desire, and due to the experience of desubjectivisation that it implies. It is *jouissance* associated with the death drive, unbinding of the drives that destructures and annihilates the desiring capacity. The enemy becomes not only the abuser, but also her own body, experienced with shame and even depreciation. It is an abused body that "deserves" punishment for having made her feel excitation in spite of herself, in an uncanny diversification of the ego. As if the girl were to say, "It didn't happen to me; it happened to my body . . ." An unmetaphorised excitation, pure cathexis, mixed with anxiety, but excitation all the same. The damage is made flesh . . . in the body. The girl consequently feels disqualified, subjected to an experience not experienced as her own.

I consider that, in this clinical work, the analyst's job is not just to lift repression in order to encourage memory and remembering. As Viderman (1970) suggests, the analyst's task is not to reveal a hidden meaning, but to construct a meaning that never formed previous to the analytic relation. In the words of Green (1990), the analyst forms an absent meaning. The analyst creates the conditions necessary to enable traumatic experience to be qualified, thought about, experienced, and spoken about, beyond historical truth but close to experiential truth in its perceptive quality.

The discourse of trauma, as Davoine (1998) points out, is always carried by someone desubjectivised by knowledge inscribed in the body, to the point that it suspends both attribution judging as well as existence judging. When time is stopped, it is because a subject is needed in order to have time, and in order to have a subject and, therefore, repression, a succession of signifiers is necessary. In the case of trauma, the chain of signifiers is interrupted, and it is precisely at this place that time is stopped, awaiting a new signifier.

A patient, thirty-five years old, a professional woman, married, with a six-year-old boy, tells me after the first interviews, in a broken voice, babbling, barely audible, that this is the first time she is able to talk about incest she suffered from her father when she was aged between seven and twelve years old. She said, "I had to construct something in my life; if not I was afraid I would break down; only now can I talk."

Might the devilish monster of traumatic experience appear in the form of the camel's question, "What do you want?" in the novel by the French author, Cazotte (1994), when it queries the fear-struck and also fascinated subject. Like Cazotte's devil in this novel, the devilishly traumatic changes shapes, maintaining great ambiguity. Traumatic experience sometimes frightens but sometimes fascinates. Whether springing from fascination or terror, the effect is the same: muteness. "Small sorrows are loquacious, great ones are mute," as Seneca said (quoted by Montaigne, 1992, p. 8, translated for this edition).

The person risks becoming an enunciate, deprived of enunciation. Even in some cases in which the person is able to speak compulsively of the traumatic experience, sometimes without modesty, this discourse is silenced, or, rather, is full of empty words.

In this case, the person is left flabbergasted, trapped in the seduction or terror of traumatic experience, not knowing what to do with it. The subject appears, in the best of cases, when the person is able to take responsibility for doing something different from what was experienced, by de-identifying from this traumatic experience.

At the centre mentioned above, the mother of an adolescent girl followed up in psychotherapy as a consequence of incest, who herself had experienced incest, came to the first interview, and when she introduced herself, instead of giving her name, said, "I am the incested woman." The traumatic experience became her identifying introduction instead, declining her identity with her own name. She "was" this enunciate. The damage suffered becomes installed as the paradoxical encysted marrow of an identity emptied of subjectivity. It is similar to what Benyakar (2005) calls the introduct, that is, something that remains encysted in the psychic apparatus without representative value. The person "is" the traumatic experience suffered. The person becomes the negative of his or her true subjectivity, oscillating between stifled muteness and Munch's scream, not finding words to tear this suffering out of the interstices of the person's being.

Sometimes, muteness in one language is unshackled in discourse that uses a different language, this passage through language called foreign perhaps facilitating verbal expression. If the subject is to verbalise suffering, to find his or her own voice, the person sometimes calls upon other languages. Far removed from the drive quality implicit in the mother tongue, they are able to express and say in an oblique way what, in the mother tongue, due to excess or deficiency, cannot be put into words: a way to produce languages according to his or her desire, that is, languages of desire.

Luciano, a patient whose mother tongue was Italian, had his analysis with me in French but sometimes used Italian, in small brushstrokes, as if his discourse were the verbalisation of an Impressionist painting. He generally used it to quote phrases he attributed to his mother, as if he had an intra-cavity relationship with her and, at the same time, would have liked to keep her at a distance by having his analysis in French. For a long time I felt that I had to listen to his few words in Italian within the totality of their drive force, and that the hospitality I gave his words in Italian was more important than the content of associations to which they referred. One day, I underscored that he used the Italian language when he was quoting phrases spoken by his mother, as if he wanted me to take care of her directly, in her native tongue. Surprised and anguished in a way I had never perceived before, he added, using a mixture of Italian and French, "Just now I realised that 'mia mamma' gave me my first kiss on the mouth." He explained that once when he was a child, his mother had passed a piece of candy from her mouth into his, that their tongues had touched in an encounter experienced as never-ending. This anguish, expressed for the first time, could not be said but in Italian, a tongue he had acquired with an excessively incestuous drive quality. It had to go through a foreign language, in this case French, in order to pacify an excessively intrusive maternal tongue. Through his analysis in French, which has a different musicality and polysemy, he could express an anguish that in his mother tongue, burning red-hot, was impossible. This patient would probably never have been able to have analysis directly in his mother tongue, hypercathected with drive quality unspeakable in his native tongue. Through the French tongue, which was also his wife's tongue, he had been able to distance himself unconsciously from the disruptive aspect of a mother tongue whose words burned him, the foreign language thereby acquiring in itself a third-party function.

The analytic function in clinical work on traumatic experience without a subject

The analytic function, after having listened to amorphous material, bits of thought, and snippets of affect, is to make a new film, as proposed by Ferro (2002). I add that it is one in which the analyst–scriptwriter may make the unspeakable of disruptive experience ("I am the incested woman") capable of figuration and, therefore, of being experienced, so that the first person singular is no longer the traumatic experience ("I am the incested woman"), but, rather, her own ego, rooted in her unconscious but freed from an alienating cystic wrapper. This requires, in Freud's words, the psychic work of construction, "by far the more appropriate description" (1937d, p. 261), shared by analysand and analyst, through which disruptive experience may finally be experienced in the first person singular.

The regression habitual in the cure leads us not so much to remembering, as is habitual in the analysis of neurotics, but to a zone of representative ambiguity in which representation becomes diffuse and is lost in a cone of shadow. To find it again, or even to produce it, would be the crossroads. However, this construction requires a previous step, which is the deconstruction of what was acting as a defence, that is, the defensive cyst of non-representation that remains split off as a pure mark awaiting meaning. Construction, in the best of cases, renders the membrane of the cyst porous and then the affect-representative of the drive breaks through the barrier, entering fluidly into circulation, without reticence, through the chain of unconscious signifiers. The hole in the chain of signifiers is then no longer an empty space aspiring to make nothingness of all meaning, but acts on a new meaning as a motor to construct meaning.

In patients subjected to traumatic experiences, the narrative ego is emptied of substance, an impersonal voice coming from far away, from some unknown memory or forgetfulness. We do not know who is speaking or to whom the person is speaking. Is it the other in me? Is it the voice of the cyst that replaced it that is speaking? The person searches endlessly for an ego; although it is always essentially dehiscent and unfinished, it may still find harmony with the subject. In order to access its own ego, connected to its conscious and unconscious affects, the narrative must be decanted from a flow of words lost in the haze of emotional–perceptive ambiguity in the defensive cyst.

Rather than a monolithic and unmoveable tower, the ego agency is like a variable geometric figure in continuous transformation, which, in spite of its polyhedron-like character, with many facets refracting its fragmentary nature, does not define the subject but, instead, places the subject on the axis of emotional responsibility.

Although the analyst is not a historian searching to re-establish historical truth of the facts but, instead, the subject's experiential truth, neither may the analyst completely abandon this search. Even though we know that the search for historical truth is destined to fail, the analyst's intervention cannot be based on a construction totally independent of what is understood of the truth of the facts. It is perhaps necessary to maintain constant tension between the search for historical truth and the mythic construction to preserve it from becoming a meticulously constructed but shaky delusion, to the point that the subject cannot get his or her footing. If not, the analytic process risks acquiring a heavy cathexis of projective suggestion on the analyst's part.

Dreams and dream production may operate then as an equivalent of remembrance. It is through dreams that the subject reappears; their perceptive intensity expresses a form of remembrance of the traumatic experience. "Free association" does not appear in the form of preconscious–conscious association, but is freed only as a transaction in dreams, a transaction that acquires the value of remembrance to the extent that the chain of dreams is taken up in the perspective of reconstruction. Sometimes, it is through dreams that the patient "remembers", and some of these scenes acquire value as memories of something that occurred.

A female patient, forty-five years old, was referred to me by her gynaecologist. His concern, not the patient's, was that she had never permitted penetration, in spite of having been married for twenty years. Her sexuality had not apparently required this form of expression, and her husband had accepted it. This impossibility would not have been a problem except that the patient did not allow any gynaecological examination that required penetration, and therefore could not have a pap test or other examinations. Obviously, we did not work on this symptom in a direct manner, but, rather, through the patient's free association. Therefore, her sexual life was not an apparent reason for concern. However, after nearly a year in therapy, a dream emerged whose manifest content was the following: "a man took her in a jeep and then in a deserted place something happened that she doesn't remember about the dream". In her associations, she recalls this man who was a friend of the family, and that one day when she was small, and although she had been in bed with fever, her mother, in her father's absence, had allowed him to take her for a ride in his jeep.

Now, in her adult's eyes, it seemed strange that her mother had accepted something as unusual as letting this man take her for a ride when she was feverish. She remembers a blanket covering her back, but what I am interested in highlighting is not so much the dream images or her associations, so evocative in themselves, but the intense feeling of suffocation and crushing she felt in her body in the dream, a feeling that was not associated with any image but whose intensity managed to wake her, deeply anguished.

Based on this dream and from the associations that followed, we "reconstructed" what might have happened, that is, the abuse by this man of which she has no memory. Her feeling in her body and her deep anguish acted, in my opinion, as a trigger to give meaning to her persistent rejection of penetration. Some part of what was disruptive had left a traumatic trace in her, so potentially painful that it led her to absent herself as a subject of pain, an extreme way to avoid it, until, through this and subsequent dreams, we were able to reconstruct what she probably suffered. When she told her husband the dream and what we had proposed as a hypothesis, he said that he was not surprised, since he had always thought she had suffered some type of abuse. Her difficulty in remembering the fact was associated, in my opinion, not only with the abuse itself, which probably occurred, but to her feeling of orphanhood due to her mother's lack of care; this was an unspeakable pain that lacerated her. Perhaps she preferred to disappear as the subject of abuse, even at the cost of her symptom, rather than to re-experience the iterated pain in her life of orphanhood due to the absence of a mother with her function of protection and caring that every child deserves.

Other situations had made her experience the pain of this absence, as, for example, when she was about eight years old, she used to have breakfast alone before going to school. For some time she went to school tipsy, because she began to drink vermouth without eating, which the school finally detected, alerting the family. Her father worked at night and was never present at breakfast time. Many other painful childhood memories emerged, but the most painful had been her actual experience of having been practically "handed over" to a person everybody referred to as "the crazy man". This person in real life finally committed suicide.

In this patient it was not so much the image of the dream, but, rather, the intensely experienced bodily feeling that was triggered and operated as an "unremembered" memory at the preconscious–conscious level.

It is as if the regressive current of the psychic apparatus during sleep functioned to trigger an old perception, neither worked through nor integrated, an unmetabolised perceptual force whose handling had remained as if suspended, awaiting the moment to be expressed; the figurable quality of the affect-representative in the dream as a substitute for the unthinkable.

We know that in dreams the regressive current allows stimulation of the perceptual pole, precisely the one that, as a consequence of disruptive experience, cannot be expressed spontaneously: it requires a construction.

However, reconstruction or construction is always approximate. As Freud stated about reconstructions (1937d, p. 260), they "can often reach only a certain degree of probability". Now, if the construction is the result of a vector of forces determined by the search for perceptual truth of the facts and the mythical construction of the scene undergone but not experienced by the subject, how do we validate the interest of this construction?

We know, as Freud highlights (1937d), that it is neither rejection nor conscious validation by the patient that enables us to infer how well grounded the proposed construction might be. Freud considers (1937d, p. 265) that in each construction "we do not pretend that an individual construction is anything more than a conjecture which awaits examination, confirmation or rejection". He compares the attitude we should take with respect to effects of the suggested construction to a phrase spoken by a character in a comedy, *Nestroy's Farces*, who, to any question or objection, would reply only, "It will all become clear in the course of future developments" (1937d, p. 265).

This ironic analogy proposed by Freud has limits, since, obviously, not everything necessarily becomes clear in the course of analysis. As noted by Stoloff (2008), construction, like the work of dream interpretation, meets the limit of what may be known in the unconscious. Just as in dreams, in which meaning escapes us through its navel, there is something like a navel of construction that it is wise to preserve. In construction, the analyst must not pretend to have an all-embracing view of the analysand's unconscious. We would do well to accept that a remnant of unknowable meaning is always left. The challenge is not so much to find the meta-psychological foundation of the construction itself for its validation, but, rather, the mutative effect of transformation the construction may achieve *après-coup* or *a posteriori* in the analysand.

In the transference relation of patients who have suffered disruptive experiences, it is particularly advisable to be aware of all the semiotics of figuration, in particular, the intonation of discourse through which we may access the unrepresented. A changing tone of voice as what is figurable in sounds of hesitations of lacunar memory of something experienced but not represented. The voice as a signifier that, through the enunciation of its sound variants, enables it to become a word cathected with affect: it allows passage from a certain affective aphasia to subjectivised discourse and emotions that flow out like a revitalising thermal spring.

Barthes (1973), in *Le plaisir du texte* (The pleasure of the text), underscores:

> With my language I can do everything: even and especially, say nothing. I can do everything with my language but not with my body. What I hide through my language my body says. I may modulate my message, but not my voice. (p. 45, translated for this edition)

The voice, its timbre, its melody or disharmony, is the least graspable aspect of analytic listening, but sometimes it also allows us to thread together an affect and its possible representation. The subject, as the affect gradually emerges, progresses from an impersonal, lifeless, or neutral voice to speaking in a living voice. It is as if the voice were speaking for itself . . . in representation of the subject, thus acquiring all its meaning. Meaning that, as Kristeva (1988) suggests, is found in the register of semiotics.

Words and silence are inseparable in the analytic process as in poetry, but this is perhaps inherent to the genesis of all aesthetics.

From this vantage point, I allow myself to suggest that psychoanalysis, at least in clinical work, is halfway between a conjectural science and a poesis in which the subject appears increasingly in the intonation, harmonious or dissonant, of the drive scansion of the voice, in its prosody, more than in the immobile meaning of an emotionally petrified enunciate. Words become full in so far as they are able to free the concomitant affect from its enclosure.

Only the appearance of a subject that may finally experience his or her suffering would make it possible, in the words of Valéry (1960), for "the past to have a future" (p. 1526), avoiding deadly compulsion repetition or psychosomatic illness. In this sense, it is naturally not a question of modifying the facts of a traumatic past. Borges (1974a, p. 575), the great clinician of the human soul, explained in "The aleph" that, "to modify the past is not to modify just one fact, it is to cancel its consequences, which tend to be infinite" (translated for this edition).

References

Assoun, P.-L. (1999). *Le Préjudice et L'Idéal. Pour une Clinique Sociale du Trauma.* Paris: Anthropos.

Barthes, R. (1973). *Le Plaisir du Texte.* Paris: Seuil.

Benyakar, M. (2006). *Lo Disruptivo.* Buenos Aires: Biblos.

Bion, W. R. (1962). A theory of thinking. *International Journal of Psycho-analysis, 43*: 306–310.

Borges, J. (1974a). El aleph. In: *Obras Completas* (pp. 533–629). Buenos Aires: Emecé.

Borges, J. (1974b). El hacedor. In: *Obras Completas* (pp. 779–854). Buenos Aires: Emecé.

Botella, S., & Botella, C. (1992). Le statut métapsychologique de la perception et l'irreprésentable. *Revue française de psychanalyse, 56*: 437–457.

Cazotte, J. (1994). *Le Diable Amoureux.* Paris: Spadem.

Davoine, F. (1998). El discurso analítico del trauma. Seminar transcribed from recording, given at the Ministry of Health, Department of Mental Health, Province of Buenos Aires, Argentina.

Ducrot, O. (1984). *Le Dire et le Dit.* Paris: Minuit.

Duras, M. (1964). *Le Ravissement de Lol V. Stein.* Paris: Gallimard.

Ferenczi, S. (1984). Reflexiones sobre el traumatismo. In: *Obras Completas* (pp. 545–563). Madrid: Espasa-Calpe.

Ferro, A. (2002). *El Psicoanálisis como Literatura y Terapia.* Buenos Aires: Lumen.

Freud, S. (1912–1913). *Totem and Taboo, S. E., 13.* London: Hogarth.

Freud, S. (1937d). Constructions in analysis. *S. E., 23*: 257–269. London: Hogarth

Freud, S. (1939a). *Moses and Monotheism. S. E., 23*: 7–132. London: Hogarth.

Green, A. (1990). *La Folie Privée.* Paris: Gallimard.

Kristeva, J. (1988). La parole déprimée. In: *La Voix, Colloque d'Ivry* (pp. 35–39). Paris: Lysimaque.

Moreno, J. (2002). *Ser Humano*. Buenos Aires: Zorzal.

Pessoa, F. (2002). *Libro del Desasosiego* [Book of Disquiet], S. Kovadloff (Trans.). Buenos Aires: Emecé.

Pirandello, L. (1993). *Sei personaggi in cerca d'autore*. Milano: Tascabili Newton.

Press, J. (2008). Construction avec fin, construction sans fin. *Revue française de psychanalyse, 82*: 1269–1337.

Quignard, P. (1998). *Vie Secrète*. Paris: Gallimard.

Roussillon, R. (1995). Métapsychologie des processus et la transitionnalité. Rapport au Congrès des Psychanalystes de Langue Française. *Revue française de psychanalyse, 59*: 1351–1519.

Seneca (undated). *Hippolyte, II*, 3, quoted by Montaigne, *Les Essais*. Paris: Arlès, 1992.

Stoloff, J.-C. (2008). Les constructions en analyse: conviction, vraisemblance et changement. *Revue française de psychanalyse, 82*: 1533–1541.

Tesone, J.-E. (2005). Incesto: el cuerpo robado. *Revista IDE, Brazilian Society of Psychoanalysis of San Pablo, 41*: 107–114.

Tesone, J.-E. (2009). *A fantasia e o simbólico na cura: do nao representável ao simbolizável*. Brasilia: Sociedade de Psicanálise de Brasilia.

Valéry, P. (1960). *Oeuvres*. Paris: Pléiade.

Viderman, S. (1970). *La Construction de l'Espace Analytique*. Paris: Denoël.

Winnicott, D. W. (1974). La crainte de l'effondrement. *Nouvelle Revue de Psychanalyse, 11*: 57–63.

CHAPTER THREE

The dynamics between "the internal bad mother" and the construction of the "bad child"*

Emilce Dio Bleichmar

> "There is no such a thing as an infant ... the infant and the maternal care together form a unit"
>
> (Winnicott, 1965, p. 39)

Introduction

The aim of this chapter is to describe some aspects of the inner world of mothers regarding their children and establish links between what psychoanalytic practice has allowed us to learn about maternal subjectivity and the descriptions given by empirical studies on early dyadic interaction. I explore a particular, but fairly frequent, mental state in many mothers analysed: a permanent, lurking feeling that they do not comply with the ideal mother model, that they cannot be "a good enough mother".

* This chapter draws on the following conference presentation: Dio Bleichmar, E. (2013). Mother–child deregulation. The internal "bad mother" complex of the mother. IPA 48th International Psychoanalytical Congress Panel: Dio Bleichmar, E., & Schejtman, C. (2013) *Mother–child Affective Regulation, Infant Self Regulation–Deregulation and Symbolic Play* (Praga).

This clinical finding raises several questions. Are these women, and perhaps women in general, prone to developing a severe superego when they become mothers? Is this superego based only on the ambivalent relationship with their own mothers, on their aggressiveness towards their pre-oedipal or oedipal mothers? Or is it also based, in addition to historical factors, on specific factors: on how maternity is culturally sanctioned in the time of the actual maternity?

The motivational caring system, which has been differentiated from the attachment system (George & Solomon, 1999), biologically – by means of oxytocin – prepares a woman to care for her baby. Contact with a helpless, suffering human being is a source of anxiety and fears that are characteristic of this early period – fear of not being able to keep the baby alive, fear of not being able to love him or her enough, fear that the child and his or her physical and emotional condition – constitute an ongoing test for "good mothers".

In the scientific literature, among health care professionals and in the media, mothers and their behaviour are constantly under scrutiny. This results in the paradox that the greater the information, the greater the obligation and, therefore, the greater feeling of self-persecution.

Besides the model of the ideal mother whom they had hoped to personify, the unconscious fantasy of being a bad mother can be a source of constant uneasiness that many mothers have to regulate in each of their intersubjective exchanges with their babies.

All these components make mothers prone to developing particularly severe, punitive forms of superego. In turn, this tends to generate a variety of strong defence mechanisms, affecting their capacity for "good enough" emotional regulation, thus interfering with their reflective capacity with their babies (Fonagy et al., 1991, 2002)

What happens in a woman's subjectivity when she becomes a mother?

The experience of motherhood has the potential to evoke representations of an archaic world and its object relations at two different levels of processing: symbolic and procedural. The desire and resolve to be a "good enough mother" are rarely absent from conscious subjectivity.

Even in conditions of maximum stress, many mothers tend to give priority to care of the infant over other pressing situations. However, when each interaction is observed – each interaction being the current focus of much empirical research on the early dyad – it is usually categorised as disruptive behaviour on the part of the mother.

Such disruption is documented in a considerable number of micro-analytic observations. Beebe and colleagues (1997), using social face-to-face exchange, examine patterns of mother–infant interaction and their relevance for the pre-symbolic origins of self and object representation. Tronick (1989) describes the micro-regulatory social–emotional process of communication that generates (or fails to generate) dyadic intersubjective states of shared consciousness. Lyons-Ruth and colleagues (2005) study the "hostile/helpless" profile considered to be present in mothers of children who have experienced loss and trauma. Schejtman and co-authors (2012), in a longitudinal study of dyadic interaction, show that "when adults are less reflective, they can probably be less empathic or somewhat intrusive. This deregulation may bring disruptions that hinder the construction or greater symbolic complexity in the playing scene" (p. 8).

Do the mothers realise that they are interfering or are not sufficiently warm, or that their emotional responses are late, or that they are invasive and emotionally deregulate the infant? Do they comprehend that emotional ambivalence is almost the rule? Are they able to tolerate negative feelings towards their infants?

It is mostly mothers who ask for a consultation for their children. Yet, when they do so, few of them accept that they might have had a role in the child's difficulties. Implicitly, the analyst is someone who might criticise them, and it is, therefore, usual for them not to reveal pertinent information.

Clinical material

Manuela has not been sleeping since the birth of her child, Mateo, who is now two years and eight months old, who also has serious difficulties going to bed. After several interviews with the child, Manuela finally tells me about her constant state of anxiety with some acute crises; at no time does she establish a link between her sleeplessness and the child's difficulty; Mateo is over-excited and alert in the evenings and she does not know how to calm him and her anxiety takes the form of irritability and a certain rejection of him. Does Manuela fall within the hostile/helpless mother category in the Lyons-Ruth and colleagues (2005) classification because her insecurity/helplessness is clear when she has to manage the child?

The analytic work with Manuela (who frequently came to sessions with her mother) allowed her unnamed anxiety to take shape. She had a good life background and had never imagined she might not be a good mother. The narcissistic injury and feeling of guilt came to the surface to give content to the permanent state of anxiety. There was no doubt that her responses to the child were sometimes inattentive and irritable, and that she sometimes made up for the distance with excessive contact. She was very up-to-date with the literature and programmes on child rearing. She came from a Catholic family and had many siblings. Her expectation of being an ideal mother had been shattered. She used a wide range of arguments and rationalisations (based on scientific information on the temperament and genetics of her husband's family) which allowed her to hold at bay a feeling of failure and confusion regarding the revolution that motherhood had brought to her life as an independent woman. This finding had plunged her into a sea of guilt that she had hidden for two and a half years – at night with persistent insomnia, during the day with drowsiness that makes her disconnected and inattentive, overwhelmed by child care.

Schejtman and colleagues (2012) conducted a longitudinal study of the dyadic mother–child relationship during the first five years of life. Data from this study described one mother, Rita, who was found to be too intrusive, leaving no room for her son to develop at the age of six months. At four years of age, he has not yet learnt to talk clearly. In her responses to the Parental Development Interview (PDI, Slade et al., 2005), she was evaluated as having a low reflective function that did not allow her to gain access to conflicting content and to the ambivalence that was illustrated by her disconnection and denial of such conflict. The mother's absence of recognition of how these denied feelings can negatively affect the child offers the key to exploring the scale that helps us to determine the quality of the reflective function.

Let us observe the interviewer asking this mother some questions from the PDI:

Interviewer: Do you ever feel angry as a mother?
Rita: As a mother?

Interviewer: Yes, as a mother.
Rita: Well, I don't know. Sometimes I find those temper tantrums or whims irritating?
Interviewer: Have you ever felt guilty as a mother?
Rita: No, not usually.

This strong denial contrasts with the answers given by María, the mother of Federico, aged four, whom we see in a video in an affectionate, creative, playful exchange with his mother. The irritations of maternity are accepted by María without any resistance and she achieves a high score in the evaluation of reflective functioning.

Interviewer: Do you ever feel angry as a mother?
María: Yes, I get angry, but maybe it's not exactly angry. I get angry to the extent that I think, "What's the matter with this child? How long is this going to last? When will he get over it?"
Interviewer: Do you ever feel guilty as a mother?
María: Yes, sometimes. That's what I've been feeling recently.

Another clinical vignette

Leticia is very worried about her three-year-old daughter, Cristina, who watches her and understands everything but does not talk. At the nursery school, they have recommended that the mother seek help in case this is selective mutism. She is an articulate, well-rounded woman with excellent family relationships, satisfied with her career and driven crazy by motherhood. She says of Cristina not talking that "There's something wrong with this child." The case study and analytic work with this mother led to recognition of a powerful mechanism of dissociation and the construction of her daughter as "a bad girl". The dominant explanation in Leticia's mind was that her daughter did not love her and that she was not important for her daughter.

The focus of interpretation was that the child undoubtedly did love her, needed her, and wanted to interact with her as much as she had wanted to be needed and loved when she was young. This understanding not only had value for interactive healing and for removing the mother's projection of the assumed aggressiveness and distancing of the child from her, but also dissolved the unconsciously feared representation, that of her identity as a bad mother.

This unconscious fantasy torments any woman, whatever her history, and we note its increasing frequency in the subjectivity of twenty-first century mothers who are subject to more and more information on how to be an excellent mother.

This leads us to the following question. Have we built theories about the persecutory anxieties that are generated by destructive fantasies in infants without taking into account the persecutory anxiety generated in the mother by the maternal superego, as well as the powerful defences built to maintain the good mother ideal? The maternal superego generates defences to avoid narcissistic suffering because motherhood constitutes a key component of the ego ideal of any woman, and the risk of losing this identification unconsciously torments them. The dominant, unconscious representation of the feared identity could give rise, in line with the personality structure, to defensive forms that disturb the capacity for emotional regulation.

Perfectionist mothers who blame their children, who project their own difficulties on their children, might distance themselves and can become indifferent. This was the case with Isabel, the mother of Beatriz, a very temperamental girl who was born with an agenesis of one ureter. Isabel had prepared herself with dedication and care for motherhood but when her child cried with pain, she despaired. Her husband calmed the infant much better than she did, and Isabel gradually detached herself from her daughter.

Archaic roots, or giving voice to current activity?

Works in the psychoanalytic literature on the female superego (Jacobson, 1976; Lax, 1992) focus on the castration complex and the equivalence of the mother's place to that of the father as the figure who punishes incestuous desires.

The incest taboo and prohibitions are key topics in psychoanalytic theory and relate to both genders but, with regard to the "ethics of care" and the abandonment of children, there is no doubt about the universality and strength of women's superego.

Although there are few studies on the role played by motherhood in women's guilt feelings, in the literature there are many categories that place the blame on mothers, such as mothers who are described as phallic, frozen, or schizophrenogenic (Dio Bleichmar, 2006).

Maternal superego

When a woman becomes a mother, what operates in her is a normative superego that is very different to that of the Freudian superego. The maternal superego is based on constant reaffirmation that she is doing things right with her child, a sort of manual of ideal feelings and procedures that real interaction refutes constantly. In her brilliant paper, Bernstein (1983) reflected the view that the superego is gendered and the girl places a sense of object-relatedness and self-worth in moral values on connectedness with others, on interpersonal relatedness, and gives relatively less weight to moral abstractions. Motherhood becomes one of the early cores of the female ego ideal, and one of the contents and objectives of her narcissistic system, providing self-esteem and efficacy to her representation of being female.

Bernstein (1983), Dahl (2002), and Tyson (1994) propose a specifically "feminine" superego which functions to sustain a sense of object-relatedness and self-worth by preserving in fantasy the relationship to the idealised pre-oedipal mother. Are women perhaps particularly vulnerable to the development of a harsh "primitive" superego when they become mothers? Is this just a re-updating of childhood conflicts, of the early superego described by Melanie Klein, or is it that the lingering internal malaise based in "the bad internal mother" developed in response to the threat posed by the conflicts and emotional reactions with her baby? As stated by Dahl, "it should be understood as an effort by the mind, in the present, to give voice to current activity" (2002, p. 4).

This mandate of the superego is constant throughout the life of many women with regard to motherhood, and conflict arises in the process of real life performance. Whether or not mothers build sound defences against constant self-criticism and self-evaluations of their own maternal superego will depend on their tolerance of conflict. The focus of the superego defences is an attempt to ward off loss of love and this lasting conflict interferes with maternal activities and warm child care (Dio Bleichmar, 2012).

Bernstein maintains that the strength of the superego refers to the efficiency with which its content is regulated. It was perhaps in this regard that Freud believed he saw weakness in the female superego, and we could perhaps link this to the conflicts that are inherent in female identity: very maternal, but not very womanly, very womanly, but not very maternal, very much an executive, but not very womanly, very maternal and no career at all (Eliacheff & Heinich, 2002). Conflict, renouncement, and guilt are always present in female subjectivity. "Women are more likely to experience conflict in choosing which of the contents will be given dominance, and they are far more likely to experience guilt (no matter what their choice)" (Bernstein, p. 189).

Après-coup *reconstruction of childhood experience*

Models of linear developmental progression pose particular pitfalls for psychoanalytic theory. The notion that the nodal events and associated conflicts specific to the developmental process might involve the erroneous assumption that the developmental process of analysis simply recapitulates the process of development, and that events and fantasies are strictly correlated.

Dahl's (2002) views are in agreement with those presented here:

> Our psychoanalytic knowledge does not reveal the developmental processes, dilemmas, and solutions as they were encountered by our analysand at an earlier age. Material presented by a particular patient during a session that, at manifest level, is replete with representations and fantasies about the archaic mother does not shed light on the actual "at the time" experience. (p. 16)

She also stated,

> The appearance of the maternal voice in intrapsychic conflict does not necessarily represent the presence of a primitive harsh superego. It is possible that some women more frequently give voice to current aspects of their inner world and its conflicts by employing representations of the archaic mother and the tie to her. (p. 15)

Bassin (1996) noted the "(c)entral importance of developmental transformation in which representations and modes of representation may be employed in new ways in attempts to solve dilemmas other than the original ones".

What we can understand is how these representations are used in the present within the mind of a particular patient. That is, these representations do not constitute windows on the past, but, rather, are attempts by the present mind to represent processes occurring in the present moment.

"We may still want to ask why representations of the archaic mother are being employed at this time. What functions do these representations serve? Are they serving to represent desires, fears, defences or superego activity?" (Dahl, 2002, p. 16).

If we were to listen with empathetic understanding to these mothers who are overloaded with feelings of persecution and fears they cannot confess (given the implicit mandate that they must love their children), the sad destiny of intergenerational transmission of the pathology can be interrupted. We could indicate to them how normal such mismatches are in most dyadic relations (Tronick, 1989), and that mismatches in communication can be dealt with and repaired.

Conclusions

The fantasy of the "bad internal mother" depends on at least three factors:

1. Awareness of the baby's helplessness and suffering, and identification with this state
2. The narcissistic component of identification with the maternal ego ideal
3. The influence of cultural ideals

The end result will depend on the strength of each of these components, and so the maternal superego is neither purely biological nor purely narcissistic nor purely transsubjective or cultural. It derives from many sources that threaten the mother's capacity to regulate emotional and caring relations with the child.

References

Bassin, D. (1996). Beyond the he and the she: toward the reconciliation of masculinity and femininity in the postoedipal mind. *Journal of the American Psychoanalytic Association, 44*: 157–190.

Beebe, B., Lachmann, F., & Jaffe, J. (1997). Mother–infant interaction structures and presymbolic self and object representations. *Psychoanalytic Dialogues, 7*: 133–182.

Bernstein, D. (1983). The female superego: a different perspective. *International Journal of Psychoanalysis, 64*: 187–201.

Dahl, K. (2002). In her mother's voice. Reflections on "femininity" and the superego. *Psychoanalytic Study of the Child, 57*: 3–23.

Dio Bleichmar, E. (2006). The place of motherhood in primary femininity. In: A. M. Alizade (Ed.), *Motherhood in the Twenty-First Century* (pp. 73–83). London: Karnac.

Dio Bleichmar, E. (2012). Modalidades del vínculo temprano como factor protector de los trastornos mentales. *VII Jornada Científica: Prevención y Detección Precoz en Psiquiatría del Niño y del Adolescente*. Fundación Alicia Koplowitz. Hospital General Universitario Gregorio Marañón. Madrid.

Eliacheff, C., & Heinich, N. (2002). *Mères-Fille, Une Relation Á Trois*. Paris: Albin Michel.

Fonagy, P., Gergeley, G., Jurist, E., & Target, M. (2002). *Affect Regulation, Mentalization and the Development of the Self*. New York: Other Press.

Fonagy, P., Steele, M., Steele, H., Moran, G., & Higgitt, A. (1991). The capacity for understanding mental status: the reflective self in parent and child and its significance for security of attachment. *Journal of Infant Mental Health, 12*: 201–218.

George, C., & Solomon, J. (1999). Attachment and caregiving: the caregiving behavioral system. In: J. Cassidy & P. Shaver (Eds.), *Handbook of Attachment: Theory, Research, and Clinical Applications* (pp. 649–670). New York: Guilford Press

Jacobson, E. (1976). Ways of female superego formation and the female castration conflict. *Psychoanalytic Quarterly, 45*: 525–538.

Lax, R. (1992). A variation on Freud's theme in "A Child is Being Beaten"—mother's role: some implications for superego development in women. *Journal of the American Psychoanalytic Association, 48*: 455–475.

Lyons-Ruth, K. Yellin, C., Melnick, S., & Atwood, G. (2005). Childhood experiences of trauma and loss have different relations to maternal unresolved and hostile/helpless states of mind on the AAI. *Attachment & Human Development, 5*: 330–352.

Schejtman, C., Huerin, Y., & Duhalde, C. (2012). A longitudinal study of dyadic and self affective regulation and its link with maternal reflective functioning along the first 5 years of life. *World Association for Infant Mental Health*, www.waimh.org/.

Slade, A., Grienenberg, J., Bernbach, E., Levy, D., & Locker, A. (2005). Maternal reflective functioning, attachment, and the transmission gap: a preliminary study. *Attachment & Human Development, 7*: 283–298.
Tronick, E. (1989). Emotions and emotional communication in infants. *American Psychologist, 44*: 112–119.
Tyson, P. (1994). Bedrock and beyond: an examination of the clinical utility of contemporary theories of female psychology. *Journal of the American Psychoanalytic Association, 42*: 447–467.
Winnicott, D. W. (1965). The theory of parent–infant relationship. In: *The Maturational Process and the Facilitating Enviroment* (pp. 37–55). London: Hogarth Press.

CHAPTER FOUR

Secrets and revelations: vicissitudes of the maternal function

Cândida Sé Holovko

In this chapter, I revisit the notion of maternal function as proposed by the École de Paris, believing that this approach expands the possibilities of reflection on psychopathology that have had an impact on psychoanalytic clinical work today. I am also concerned about the lack of promotion of this concept in Latin America.

I discuss some episodes of the psychoanalytic process of a twenty-five-year-old woman, who has been bulimic since the age of fifteen. In this particular case, I try to reflect upon the consequences of an insufficiency of the maternal function and how it was possible for the analysis to widen the psychic space of this analysand, whose suffering was so intense that she could barely grasp it, due to living in a kind of forced exile. I stress particularly the moments where the compulsive bulimic behaviour as a prime defence is replaced and transformed into a more neurotic narrative, that is, psychic experiences, where representations and linked affects appear. I also propose some hypotheses about the vicissitudes of the maternal function in this particular case. The notion of maternal function that I use tries to account for the creation of a psychic apparatus capable of managing the impacts of existence. It also provides an aid to understanding of the psychopathologies that might occur through deficits in the foundations of this introjective function.

It is relevant to refer to the concept of maternal function as developed by Fain (2001–2002), who enriched and deepened the concept initially developed by Pierre Marty, who mostly emphasised the libidinal cathexes that the mother provides for each of the functional systems of the infant (both psychic and somatic) regulating the operation of excitations that affect the child. Fain broadens the notion of maternal function when marking the importance of an early triangular situation (the baby, the mother, and the not-mother, that is, another in whom the mother invests libido) in the origin of the processes of subjectivation. This gives a bigger emphasis to the triangulation that is present ever since the origins of object interaction.

The concept of maternal function covers libidinal investments towards the infant and what the mother disposes to the infant that will lead the way to the autoeroticisms and the constitution of hallucinatory processes, which are the bedrock for the processes of symbolisation/representation.

According to Smadja (2010):

> This discontinuity of maternal investments is similar to M. Fain's concept of the woman alternately mother and lover, at the time when she withdraws the maternal investments from the child to invest in the father erotically, withdrawal that leads to a censorship from the lover, creating the mark within which the identifying aptitudes of the child to the mother's desire can be deployed. (p. 94)

This means that when the baby identifies him or herself with the mother who desires what the father can offer, it opens a path to the early feminine identification in both sexes, and when he or she identifies with this "other" desired by the mother, it will favour the masculine identification, thus creating the grounds for the psychic bisexuality, as Fain (1971) has shown in his article "Prelude to phantasy life" and which Tabacof (2013) highlights regarding the fact that the pulsional development of the infant will be "marked by the phantasmatic richness, by the psychic defence mechanisms and the capacity of sublimation, as he will be apt for regressive movements and have access to passivity, so crucial to psychic life" (personal communication).

However, distortions in the introjection of the object with maternal function may occur due to deficiencies in primary relationships, marked either by a highly invasive and excessive presence, or by a feeling of abandonment from absence, or, furthermore, by the disruptive discontinuity, which would lead to failure in libidinisation and the para-excitation system, leading to what Tabacof (2013) states in terms of traumatic lineage:

> These patients' refusal of passivity can be understood as a consequence of the intense fear of falling into an endless abyss, as a result of the absence of an internal object to hold on to . . . the Ego becomes the owner of the game, external reality becomes the foreground . . . compulsive behaviours are established as an anti-traumatic defence to fight the appearance of the crude material coming out of these non-symbolised residues, that could not be integrated into the repressed unconscious. . . . Repetition compulsion because there is no phantasmatic correlate to support it . . . due to a failure in the attempt of pulsion intrication; thus the subject is kept prisoner in the circle of repetition. (personal communication about the work presented in Rio de Janeiro, translated for this edition)

From the patient's story—I will call her Nicole—we can detect an undifferentiated and conflicted relationship with a mother who is felt to be invasive, dictatorial, and hypercritical, and a father who is experienced as submissive in relation to this omnipotent wife, a father who removes himself from participating in family life. These dynamics are commonly seen in patients with eating disorders.

It is well known that eating disorders are nowadays presented as old pathologies in new garments since they have been described for centuries. According to data from Ambulin (www.ambulin.org.br), a centre of reference in Brazil for pathologies such as these (Hospital of the São Paulo Medical School), around ninety to ninety-five per cent of the cases occur in teenage girls (mostly anorexics) and between twenty- to thirty-year-olds (mostly bulimics). In men, the percentage is over the ten per cent threshold, which represents a 100% increase in the past five years. The majority of these disorders in men also occur in adolescents between thirteen and eighteen years of age. We ask what this significant increase might mean. This surprising result of an exponential increase in eating disorders in men brings to mind André's (2013) paper, "Male homosexuality in the analytic treatment", where he approaches, among other ideas, the psycho-socio-cultural consequences of sexual liberation that started in the 1920s and intensified in the 1960s; he affirms that the sexual "revolution" did not only free the woman in women, but also in men, too. The most recent wave of emancipation has to do with sexual choice, the freedom to desire the other or the same (homos) sex (André, 2013). We know that the eating disorders that affect women are mainly the result of failures in the early mother–infant relations, especially of the vicissitudes of the separation and individuation of the mother–daughter processes. Could the early mother–son separation and individuation processes be changing as well?

Theories explaining eating disorders have undergone additions and changes over time since Freud, who primarily identified in these problems the expression of a regression of the genital sexuality to orality. Initially, they were thought of as libidinal conflicts with symptoms of hysterical organisation; however, now we have started acknowledging, due to the severity of these behaviours, signs of great internal destructiveness more closely connected to issues of the pathologies of limits: fragility of narcissistic bases and problematics of primary identity.

In the case of bulimia, there is a desperate attempt to incorporate food/mother-object to fill the void of an internal object. In this precise sense, the subject is looking for an external object which, when incorporated, becomes toxic because it is filled with oral sadistic drives directed to the object, and the intrusion of contents that do not belong to the patient, which will trigger an urgent need to expel them.

Revealing secrets

Nicole has a secret. She has kept it for ten years, like a talisman, a triumph (Bidaud, 1998), allowing her to have a sense of power, of dominion, with which she is pleased, but, at the same time, it is endured as if it were a curse. She decides to begin sharing it in analysis—three sessions a week using the couch—with expectations of leaving her solitary confinement. For the first time, and at the risk of exposing her vulnerabilities, she confides that, since the age of fifteen, she has had bulimic symptoms, which are expressed by an uncontrollable compulsion to eat absolutely everything in her reach, and the ensuing overwhelming desire to vomit. Initially, the expulsion of food was induced by a finger in her throat, which was slowly replaced by automatic vomiting. It is a compulsion that has been there for ten years and that is repeated two to three times a day, a deep secret kept hidden from anyone she knows. It is possible that the right to possess this secret (Aulagnier, 1976) has for many years been an attempt to ensure a certain amount of autonomy of her internal space and object relations, especially a self-sufficiency regarding the mother figure. Aulagnier (1976) suggests that the existence of the secret may reveal a vital part of psychic functioning.

Problems with eating began when Nicole was twelve years old with a compulsion towards types of food that caused her much embarrassment on account of her weight gain. During her teenage years, Nicole felt dull and very shy, and she could not stand the sight of men, including her own father. At that time, she began to menstruate, but did not tell anyone because the irrefutable proof that she had a woman's body provoked in her enormous revulsion. Due to the insistence of a fifteen-year-old boy, she became his girlfriend and they started having sex; simultaneously, the bulimic symptoms appeared, in which vomiting, according to Nicole, had the function of making her thinner. It seems she had a counterpart period of anorexia when she was trying to eliminate her feminine form (she could not stand her breasts and buttocks, and could not bear the thought of getting pregnant) and remained some time without menstruating. It was a clear rejection of her mother and all that was feminine in her, for Schaeffer (2008, p. 57) these girls become self sufficient and "*phallicisée*" by their anorexia.

She chose to attend college in another province and a specialist course even further from her parents' house, but ended up choosing the same career as her mother. Despite her attempts to put the object at a distance, the geographical isolation did not prevent Nicole from continuing to be merged with the original maternal object.

Brusset (1989) describes the passionate and paradoxical dimension of the relationship of the anorexic/bulimic with her mother in that the latter represents everything that provokes horror, through a feeling of dispossession of the daughter's emotional, mental, and physical space, but who, at the same time, is the indispensable mother whose oral archaic link cannot be undone.

Nicole tells me that when she was little she was very attached to her mother's breast, and was breastfed up to six years old. When her mother left, Nicole mentions that she kept holding on to one of her bras, waiting for her to return. In this situation, we can think of a distorted introjection of the object with maternal function, as a result of excessive presence that produced, among other things, failures in the para-excitation system and difficulties in establishing a primary hallucination of the object. Thus, she was prevented from developing autoerotic activities (thumb sucking, for example), and from creating transitional objects that could help replace the primary object. The mother's bra, which is used next to the body, has here less of a transitional object function and appears more as a fetish to fill the gap of the representation of an internal object. We wonder what leads a mother to breastfeed her daughter for so many years? What is the place that the daughter occupied in the psychic dynamic of this mother?

This situation recalls clinical material described by Szwec (2013) in *Les galériens volontaires* (1989), where a mother who responded quickly to the discomfort of her baby and her increased tension offered the breast as a self-soothing measure. He showed how this repetitive behaviour of the mother eventually started off in her baby a "*neo besoin*" breastfeeding at the expense of setting up autoerotism suction. "The mother uses her son as a 'calming machine' and she becomes for him such a 'calming machine' too in a mechanised breastfeeding made independent from the satisfaction of hunger and pleasure" (p. 75, translated for this edition).

Nicole's breastfeeding until six years of age could also have favoured the creation of a neo-necessity in the baby (McDougall, 1995) when appeasing affects are experienced as unbearable. Following the same idea Bidaud, 1998, proposes a relationship with a mother-drug, a tranquilliser mother.

The relationship Nicole has with her parents, in particular her mother, is highly ambivalent. She mentions a critical, domineering mother, who does not accept differentiation and individuation. However, at the same time, Nicole complains of maternal absence, emotional void, and an immense solitude and premature autonomy. We might ponder that she complains about the deficiency of the introjection of the maternal function that could make her detach from the original object so as to create an identity. She also complains of an excessive presence of content that does not belong to her and that invades her psychosoma. Too much presence and absence—too full and too empty. Too much intake and expulsion, characterising what Miranda (2010) has called pathology of opposites. According to the author, "Mother and daughter living a passionate story, in which one can not stop nurturing the other even for a moment, because they are united by the same destiny, caught in the same body" (Miranda, 2010, p. 200). If the mother invests too much in the child, she will somehow impede auto-erotism and fantasy life. The lack of an internal object could then have disastrous consequences for the symbolic activity, as McDougall (1995) proposes about the subject.

Nicole decides to start an analysis to understand why she has avoided intimacy with others and mainly to understand what this compulsion is that makes no sense to her, a compulsion that leaves her exhausted in an infernal cycle of voracity and expulsion of food. Nicole stated, "When I ate I felt accompanied, it was a caress, but immediately I had to go and throw up. Vomiting was a relief." The paradoxical compulsion that entangled her was becoming unbearable. "My life was reduced to eating, vomiting, and work. I do not want to waste my youth; I wasted a lot of time doing it . . ."

At fifteen years of age, her parents discovered Nicole's bulimia/anorexia and took her to a psychiatrist, and it was a terrible experience for her. After that, they made a pact of silence and everything worked as though she had recovered from a passing crisis. In the relationship with her parents, she always tried to avoid talking about issues related to emotions. In one session, she said she was tired of that theatre and decided to tell her mother everything she had not told for all those years. It was a great vomiting out in which her anger was named and recognised, reminiscent of Dumet (2008).

With the analysis, a period of greater care towards her body began. I realise she seeks a continent object, non-intrusive, to strengthen her narcissistic basis, resulting in terms of countertransference in a maternal anxiety in me, a feeling that we were walking into a minefield and that I had to take the utmost care in offering only small portions of food/words to avoid her vomiting them. Nicole goes, spontaneously for the first time, to see a psychiatrist, a nutritionist, and a dentist. She finds out that she has reflux and gastritis, and that all the vomiting has destroyed the enamel that covered her teeth. Anxiety increases along with the desire to get out of that deadly circle that imprisons her.

Initially, she significantly reduces the amount of food ingested but, as time went by, she gradually tries to increase the amount of food, little by little, so as not to vomit. Now she feels horror at the thought of vomiting. Childhood memories start to emerge and we talk about how food associated with amorous experiences need not be expelled as if it were toxic intrusions into the body.

Some sessions later, feeling guilty for having been so aggressive with her mother, she begins to tell me about her dreams, which happen with increasing frequency. In one dream she is seven years old in a scene of sexual violence:

> A man shoves his hand violently inside her pants. The man was saying in a seductive voice, "*You like it, baby, of course you like it.*" She woke up terrified and with the firm belief that it had been a real abuse. Upon waking, she heard herself repeating again and again the name of a neighbour, the father of a childhood friend.

The phrase "*You like it, baby*" could be a sentence that she actually heard, or a phantasised one. It could be the expression of guilt for bodily sensations aroused by the intrusion of the adult's desire in the girl's body. We might postulate that it might be related to the confusion of mouth/vagina. The finger penetrating the vagina might be an equivalent of the nipple that is introduced indiscriminately to cover what disturbs, confused with hunger, which may have been experienced as an intrusion in the psychosoma. We recall that she was breastfed until she was six years old, so that the dream might represent real experiences of invasion not only due to excessive breastfeeding, but also as a result of possible real abuse by an adult man.

Tesone (Chapter Two) states,

> It is as if the regressive current of the psychic apparatus during sleep functioned to trigger an old perception, neither worked through nor integrated, an unmetabolised perceptual force whose handling had remained as if suspended, awaiting the moment to be expressed; the figurable quality of the affect-representative in the dream as a substitute for the unthinkable.
>
> We know that in dreams the regressive current allows stimulation of the perceptual pole, precisely the one that, as a consequence of disruptive experience, cannot be expressed spontaneously: it requires a construction. (p. 26)

In one particular session, which occurred after a week's interruption of analysis, Nicole describes an experience reminiscent of the cases of hysteria described by Freud in early psychoanalytic theory. I think we were facing a type of hysterical conversion, possibly, a movement of hysterisisation of the bulimic symptom.

Nicole goes to a work-related congress with her mother, and becomes very anxious for fear of meeting the man who had at that time awakened a strong desire in her. In her hotel room she went through something that initially seemed like a dream: suddenly, she is sitting on the bed, doing body movements like a person who is vomiting, she had her arms outstretched, hard and writhing as if having a seizure. She begins to shout very loudly, "*No, no and no*!" and cries compulsively. A colleague walks into the room and Nicole extends her arms to embrace her. The woman tries to calm her, very tenderly. Nicole speaks as if she was a child and tells her that it could not be possible, they did many bad things to her. The woman wants to know what is happening. Nicole replies, "I was very young, I was only fifteen."

When Nicole recounts all this in the session, she is surprised by the words "very young" and "fifteen". She says that while the colleague tried to calm her down, she awoke from what she considered to have been a dream and asked the woman what was going on. The woman told her what she saw and only then did Nicole realise that it was not a dream. The person escorted her to the room where her mother was, and Nicole did not mention anything so as not to worry her. She tells me she was really lucky to have been found by such a tender, sympathetic colleague.

Later that evening, she attended supper with colleagues from the congress, including the man she desired. She avoided speaking to him. Then something happened that she cannot understand: at dinner she ate everything naturally without restricting the type of food, without wondering if something would not go down well, and without overeating. She feels very surprised by the fact. After that episode, Nicole declares that she has been eating in a very natural way.

In this sequence of events, we have the opportunity to glimpse a transformation of compulsive actions from deficient psychic structures, with flaws in symbolisation expressed by bulimic acts, into a more hysterical mechanism of defence in which the act has meaning and seeks communication within a more neurotic, phantasmatic universe. We see evidence of the staging of strong drive intensity and conflict. A register of feminine seduction figured in the colleague/substitute mother, and another register of the seduction of a man who provokes desire. Could Nicole be expressing psychic bisexuality, characteristic of hysterical conflicts? Would her body movements be a mimesis of the sexual act, oral and/or genital? Would they be the expression of the conflict between desire and refusal in relation to penetration, against which she fights?

In her account, there is an estrangement with the expression, "I was very young, I was only fifteen." It could refer to two or more registers of sexual seduction: one with her boyfriend—when she first had sex at fifteen years of age—which was experienced as an act of sexual violence (the time when the first symptoms of bulimia arose), another older register, from when she was seven, possibly a real event of sexual violence with her neighbour, and also an even earlier experience of seduction, that is, the incessant intrusion of the maternal breast until six years old, which could have been experienced *après-coup* as violent abuse.

After a period of strong resentment against her parents, Nicole starts to get closer, asking for help and trying to understand them. She reveals the "hysterical conversion" episode to her mother, which provokes in her much concern and anxiety. It was at that moment that the mother told her a secret: she herself, the mother, had suffered from eating disorders in her teenage years, before she got married. She revealed for the first time to her daughter her bulimia/anorexia: usually, for a week, Nicole's mother would eat absurd amounts of food until saturation, and in the following week ate absolutely nothing, being weak to the point of fainting. The mother told her of the problems she had with Nicole's maternal grandmother, the experiences of abandonment with an extremely narcissistic mother.

Here we can note that the transgenerational distortions in the introjection of the object with maternal function occurred because of deficiencies in primary relationships: either marked by a highly invasive and excessive presence, or by a feeling of abandonment from absence.

It seems that Nicole had a register of bulimia, a compulsive act through which she reacted with her body, and a hysterical account that, in this last session, moved into the foreground. When Nicole says she now eats everything naturally, we can consider the hypothesis that what is at stake is the abandonment of the exclusive relationship breast/mother and an extension of the possibilities of incorporation. She is shocked about eating naturally again without compulsion, which makes us think she is surprised by the appearance of a more sophisticated level in her psychic experience. The acting out in Nicole's hysterical conversion also reveals a displacement of the loving maternal transference, previously towards the analyst, then to the colleague, at a time of absence from analysis.

This moment of the analysis marks a change in the way the patient treats the excitements that invade her psyche. One notes here a better capacity for linking the excitement and the qualities in the psychic processes: dream elaborations, childhood memories, expressions of desires and affections attached, connected through more neurotic symptomatology. The narration shows triangulations and investigative curiosity that express an analytic process in motion.

In this material, we are dealing with very complex clinical situations that have had a profound impact in psychoanalytic clinical work. The action of sharing experiences is more necessary than ever as part of further instrumentalisation. These winding roads can lead either to solutions with strong and deadly defensive charges (in certain configurations) or, rather, with luck and good objects, to defensive solutions that seek to expand psychic and intersubjective capacities with strong vital colouring.

References

André, J. (2013). Male homosexuality in the analytic treatment. Presentation to the COWAP meeting, Istanbul, May.

Aulagnier, P. (1976). Le droit au secret: condition pour pouvoir penser. *Nouvelle Revue de Psychanalyse, 14:* 141–157.

Bidaud, E. (1998). *Anorexia mental, Ascese, mística: Uma abordagem psicanalítica.* Rio de Janeiro: Companhia de Freud.

Brusset, B. (1989). *La relation d'objet.* Paris: Le Centurion.

Dumet, N. (2008). Agir de mort, agir de vie: quand la boulimie (se) fait rage. In: B. Chouvier & R Rouissillon (Eds.), *Corps, acte et symbolisation.* Brussels: De Boeck.

Fain, M. (1971). Prélude à la vie fantasmatique. In: *Revue Française de Psychanalyse, 35*(2-3) (pp. 291–364). Paris: PUF.

Fain, M. (2001–2002). The maternal function according to Pierre Marty. *Revue Française de Psychosomatique, 20*: 47–52.

McDougall, J. (1995). *The Many Faces of Eros: A Psychoanalytic Exploration of Human Sexuality.* New York: W. W. Norton.

Miranda, M. R. (2010). A Representação Simbólica nas Perturbações Alimentares à luz da Complexidade da Relação mãe-filha. In: A. P. Gonzaga & C. Weinberg (Eds.), *Psicanálise de Transtornos Alimentares* (pp. 199–217). São Paulo: Editora Primavera.

Schaeffer, J. (2008). Une symbolisation du sexe feminine: est-elle possible? In: B. Chouvier & R. Roussillon (Eds.), *Corps, acte et symbolisation*. Brussels: De Boeck.

Smadja, C. (2010). *La vida operatória: estudios psicoanalíticos*. Madrid: Editorial Biblioteca Nueva.

Szwec, G. (1989). *Les galériens volontaires: Essais sur les procédés autocalmats*, Paris. Presses Universitaires de France.

Szwec, G. (2013). Sobre o uso autocalmante do pavor. Presented to the 2º Psychoanalytic Psychosomatics, Rio de Janeiro, 2013.

Tabacof, D. (2013). Comments on "Sobre o uso autocalmante do pavor" by G. Szwec, presented to the 2º Psychoanalytic Psychosomatics, Rio de Janeiro, 2013.

Tesone, J.-E. (2013). ¿Dolor psíquico sin sujeto? Work presented to the Symposium de la Asociación Psicoanalítica Argentina, 2013.

CHAPTER FIVE

Bereaved families after neonatal death*

Teresa Lartigue

Introduction

In Western culture, when two individuals in a committed relationship of love and intimacy have decided to have or adopt children, it is believed that the couple is transformed into a family, the fundamental unit of the social world. In general, the family is formed as a result of the couple's life and as a typical institution of adult life. Few decisions are as significant as that of bringing children to the world, which imposes on the couple the condition of living in a triangular structure, that of the Oedipus complex, which is fundamental to the development of human beings.

At the same time, the family is the basic unit that provides the adequate resources to satisfy fundamental human needs and forms the smallest, but optimal, unit to perpetuate society. The family transmits norms and behavioural codes, myths and beliefs, language, traditions, ethical precepts, and rules about gender relationships as a

* An earlier version of this chapter was presented to the XI Latin American Intergenerational Dialogue between Men and Women, COWAP, Buenos Aires, Argentina, on September 2014: "Gender and parenting: impact on subjectivity".

couple and with other members of society. Thus, the family is a key building block with which society is formed; however, it is worth noting that there are as many modalities of the family institution as diverse cultures in the world (Vives & Lartigue, 2003). The family is also a space for the containment of psychological and somatic suffering, and it creates an environment in which the capacity for communication and thought develops (Losso, 2001).

In providing care to a considerable number of families that have suffered the loss of a child, I have come to understand in all its fullness the irreparable, and occasionally the unspeakable, features of such events, no matter the age at which the loss occurs, whether as an embryo, foetus, newborn, during the first year of life, or in any stage of life. The psychological suffering, pain, affliction, hopelessness, and sadness that this type of loss entails are inexpressible and remain throughout the years (Lartigue, 2005; Lartigue & Vives, 1994; López et al., 1997).

It is a psychological trauma—and sometimes a physical one when the mother's life is at risk—to the extent that, as mentioned by Maldonado-Durán and colleagues (2013), there are thought disturbances, a reduction in the capacity for mentalization, difficulties in affect regulation, disorganised attachment patterns, and difficulties in intersubjective relationships. Likewise, an important number of defensive functions are activated, which include: dissociative phenomena, identification with the aggressor, unexplainable states of intense anxiety, and social inhibitions in general. Other functions that are employed are the mechanisms of denial, projection, reaction formation, displacement, compensation, rationalisation, as well as the use of fantasy and wishful thinking, and projective identifications. The transgenerational can appear as well in an abrupt and violent manner.

In the context of current life expectancies, it is generally believed that children will outlive their parents and not the other way around. The aim of this chapter is to highlight the need for a long-term psychoanalytic or psychotherapeutic treatment, at least for three years (not only a crisis intervention), since the traumatic effects could lead, two or three years after the event, to a condition that attacks the mother's immunological system, where the "defences weaken" and the mother's life is at risk. Likewise, the chapter aims to promote reflection on the resources that are at play when coping with the psychological suffering as a response to an unexpected neonatal death in a family formed by the father, mother, and a daughter.

Treatment can help parents learn to live with their pain, to stop them from dying with their death, to help them assimilate the multiple vicissitudes of grieving, to deal with the problem of guilt (and its inseparable partner, the need for punishment) to the extent that it is possible, and to be able to continue with everyday life and recover the pleasure and joy of living, especially when they have other children. The treatment also aims to prevent the child who is born after the neonatal death from exhibiting the replacement child phenomenon (Cain & Cain, 1964; Lartigue & Maldonado-Durán, 1998).

Clinical vignette

Carlota is a married woman who was twenty-eight years of age when she sought psychoanalytic therapy with the aim of solving marital difficulties: if she was unable to solve them, she thought, perhaps the best option would be divorce or separation. My first impression was of meeting a bright woman, with a highly developed critical thinking capacity, who had an excellent research position, was independent and autonomous, and with a two-year-old child. Carlota is the second child of a dysfunctional family of three children, in which the father and the mother remain together despite having a very poor relationship, mainly due to financial problems. The mother's overprotection of the youngest child stands out, and this has caused innumerable family difficulties.

After fourteen months of psychoanalytic psychotherapy (fifty-minute sessions once a week) and with a flexible psychoanalytic frame in the sense of the possibility of changing appointments due to her job, which required regular travelling, Carlota proposed to finish her treatment and I agreed, since she felt there were positive changes in her life. In addition, there was a considerable improvement in the relationship with her nuclear family and with her husband, which led Carlota and her husband to plan a second pregnancy. We said goodbye when she was approximately fourteen weeks into her pregnancy, leaving the door open in case she needed therapy in the future.

Six months later, Carlota's mother telephoned to inform me that the night before, Carlota had given birth to a baby girl who died an hour after birth due to pre- and postnatal complications. Carlota's mother mentioned that Carlota wished to see me and I visited her at the hospital. I remember that, when I arrived, Carlota's depressive state was evident; she was lying down on the bed, with considerably swollen eyes because of crying, and with bleeding in the right eye, which was caused, she told me, by crying all night. She was recovering from a caesarean section carried out the night before, but, above all, she was suffering from intense post traumatic shock.

Carlota told me, "I could not sleep the night before; I was not feeling tired." After talking with her, I realised that she was terrified of sleeping because "I feared dying or reviving the moment in which my child died"; she mentioned that "while I was in surgery, and my body was open, I heard my child fighting for her life and unfortunately I could not do anything to save her, that helplessness caused me great sorrow." Carlota also mentioned that she felt tightness in her chest. Carlota did not sleep for two days after her child's death, which hindered her physical recovery. For this reason, Carlota reported that her gynaecologist gave her medication to induce sleep and prioritise her physical and emotional recovery.

From that day onwards, Carlota required daily home-based psychotherapeutic treatment for a month, since she had serious physical and emotional difficulties that limited her ability to carry out her activities as before. In those first weeks, the main challenges were, in her words, "the anxiety disorders, the lack of sleep, the irritability and considerable difficulty concentrating, which ended in a nervous breakdown" a month after the baby's death, which became apparent through an inflammation of the intercostal nerves, which were swollen to the point of not permitting normal motility and respiration. The latter required the intervention of an orthopaedics specialist who was able to treat her to reduce the inflammation.

Two months after her baby's death, Carlota said she was a "bit better physically, but with serious psychological limitations." She mentioned that her "child's loss destroyed the dreams the family and I had constructed in relation to Andrea's birth, it was an irreparable loss." She added, "On each birthday, in each picture, at each social gathering, in each child at the age Andrea would have been, I will feel her loss; I am condemned to a lifelong pain." For Carlota, it was especially difficult to see her other child, who was four years of age, undergo her little sister's death. Carlota and her husband gave this child the news the same day that the baby died. It was also especially difficult for Carlota to realise that Andrea "died because of an act of clinical negligence. I was very disappointed with the health professionals' care, the helplessness of not being able to change things hurts me, which was an additional problem in dealing with Andrea's loss."

She used to tell me that seeking the best practice, she found the worst; she had changed gynaecologist precisely because she wished to have a natural childbirth, as she had for her first child; she did some research and, through various recommendations, contacted the medical team that treated her. Carlota and I began to ask ourselves about possible circumstances that led to Andrea's death, as the result of a cardiac problem. Carlota, as a good scientist, looked for all possible causes of neonatal death on the internet, arriving at a probable cause: two days before childbirth, she had suffered from haemorrhoids and the gynaecologist had prescribed a drug. Carlota did more research and then corroborated with a specialist in cardiology and neonatology that the prescribed drug obstructed the baby's arterial duct.

In her sessions Carlota reported that being unable to work makes her lose money, opportunities, and professional development. She added, "I also can't be the mother that I used to be, my depression and sadness stops me from giving my daughter the attention that she needs, I also can't be the wife that I used to be, or the friend that I used to be." She told me that she felt "cut off from others, in an isolated emotional state that without a doubt did not take long to damage my most important relationships." Carlota reported "a marked reduction in my interest or participation in meaningful activities, a restriction of my affective life, the feeling that the future looks bleak, pessimism, and an incapacity to perform my job, and I have spent almost four months without working." With the aim of helping Carlota and her family, I recommended colleagues to her who could provide treatment to her husband and her daughter, both of whom were going through similar crises.

Carlota said, "During those times it was particularly difficult to take care of my daughter. On the one hand, she had developmental regressions that require extra care." On the other hand, Carlota's depression reduced her energy and vigour to satisfy her needs. The same occurred with her husband Alberto; Carlota felt that he "needed me more than ever but I was more indisposed than ever."

Carlota felt that she had "to start all over again, to start being a mother, a wife, to work, even to breathe again." In the first few days, she reported "having pain in everything I did, living was unbearable"; she said that breathing was painful and that she "devoted time during the day to shedding tears and getting rid of the pain." She also made reference to the difficulty of dealing with her social life after her newborn's death. Answering those phone calls from people asking whether the baby had already been born, Carlota used to reply that the baby had been born, but that, in addition to being born, the baby had also died.

Time passed and Carlota kept facing the effects of the loss, especially a constant fear that something would happen to her loved ones. Carlota mentioned that she felt that she had lost her innocence, she has had a very bitter taste of life, and nobody and nothing can fix it, and that she cannot trust the world the way she used to. She added, "I feel that a part of me died with Andrea."

Carlota mentioned that she felt an immense pain when she remembered "the caesarean section in which Andrea was fighting for her life and I was unable to do anything about it, when the doctor said that Andrea died"; also when Carlota and her husband gave the news to their little daughter. When she remembers the "only moment I had with my child, dead in my arms, I think that in that instant I experienced the saddest event that can be witnessed in nature—a mother holding her dead baby." When she looks at a picture of her family and knows that it will never be complete because her daughter is missing, when she thinks that she "did not see my child alive, I never saw her eyes open, and I will have to learn to live with a sadness that will remain all my life", she felt as if she had an incurable disease.

At the same time that Carlota was working with, and making sense of, her loss, six months after Andrea's death, Carlota and her husband planned another pregnancy. She continued her research into what she called "an accident of an inefficient health system".

The birth of Gabriela, a healthy and beautiful girl (fourteen months after Andrea's death) brought happiness, but also an immense sadness; I again saw Carlota at her home, and she could not stop crying thinking of her little Andrea. Gradually, with the help of psychotherapy, her husband's support, the support of her nuclear family and her two daughters, Carlota started recovering her maternal functions and her wish to live again. A greatly helpful technique in

Carlota's treatment was my recommendation of writing down everything that crossed her mind, as in automatic writing (Lanza Castelli, 2010). Writing at nights or in the morning gave her comfort. We said goodbye one more time.

Two years after Andrea's death (and ten months after Gabriela's birth), Carlota phoned me again in tears asking to arrange a meeting; she had found out that her husband had been unfaithful to her. In addition to working with her in individual psychotherapy and for a limited number of sessions, I recommended they seek couple therapy with a colleague, who saw them immediately. Carlota and Alberto agreed to a temporary separation and both of them began working hard to save their relationship; they realised that a significant part of their current situation was related to Andrea's death and the "symbolic death of the couple". They also realised that they loved each other deeply; they renewed their marital contract, and began living together again. We said goodbye once more.

On the third anniversary of Andrea's death, she called me again. She told me that she had been falling ill constantly and that she had had blood tests and her immune system was weak, that she was missing the group of defences that attack bacteria, and that she had scheduled an appointment with an immunologist who had recommended several tests, one of them in the USA. Carlota commented that she had a serious type of influenza, one that put her life at risk, and that she was afraid of dying, of choking, of not being able to breathe. She asked me to "please help me think about what is happening to me". We formulated some hypotheses on this matter and she added, "I think during these three years I have been punishing myself, as if a part of me was teaching myself a lesson for being a bad mother to Andrea. I can link it to dreams I have had. I think this has led me to some sort of depression. The death wish is something that must be deep inside because I have never felt it or perceived it in dreams, but now that I have felt relatively close to it because of the issue of the defences, I see that it is there deep down and that worries me a lot."

Carlota also mentions that looking back at the past three years, especially the last year and a half, she has been in very poor health, whereas before she was a very healthy child and adolescent. Regarding the influenza, she mentioned that she had had it along with the unusual symptom of not having a fever, but that she felt so unwell that she had the test done. Carlota consulted a specialist in immunology and allergies, who prescribed her drugs, complete rest, and to be kept in quarantine. Her husband was supposed to travel and had to postpone his trip because of the doctor's recommendation. For seven days she was unable to leave her house and, to her great surprise, her youngest daughter, who had "become a tyrant" (for not letting Carlota sleep at night, as she screamed "I want my mummy", and Carlota tells her "I am here, look at me I have to sleep", but the child throws a tantrum and cries), during those seven days, the child slept through the night.

Carlota says, "This is going to be my year, I am going to take care of myself, recover my health and life", but she bursts into tears and comments that she had not been able to be the mother that she used to be with her elder daughter. Regarding Gabriela, she realises that she overprotects her, that she gets very anxious and has let her child control her; all the effects that Andrea's death has had on her family had been very painful for Carlota. In the past three years, in addition to the loss and the pain, Carlota's poor health, and impact of her husband's affair, he had had to start a new job which involved being away from home three days a week. She realised that she leads "a solitary life, I had been isolated, I still have a debt from my Master's scholarship and I have overspent it by buying stuff for me and the girls, as psychological compensation, as a way of loving myself." She mentions that her husband's trips mean staying alone with the girls, and she is afraid that something could happen to them. Carlota comments that she feels a lot of tension in her life; she has worked so much, conducting projects, and she has not been paid in eight months.

In relation to a hypothesis that was developed in treatment, that her illness could be due to an unconscious sense of guilt and, consequently, a need for punishment, Carlota tells me that she had been thinking that she worked too much while she was pregnant with Andrea and that that might have been the reason she had the haemorrhoids which were the cause of taking the drug—which was wrongly prescribed. I ask her to try to think about all the self-criticism she might have because of her child's death; she says, "The effects have been overwhelming in my family, in the relationship with my husband, in the relationship with my daughters and the relationship with myself, in my health. But I am already taking action, and I would like to come to a number of sessions with you to get back on track." She says that with her youngest daughter she will not allow herself to be controlled; she realises that this happened because of her overprotection and the fear that Gabriela could die as well, but that her daughter is already in nursery school and she only cried for a few minutes during her first four days in school. Her elder daughter, on the other hand, was better, she was more sociable; Carlota realised that she was afraid to take her out to the street; both of them had been cut off from others. Carlota tells me that she realised that she was unable to deal with everything at once, and now needed to take care of herself.

In another session, Carlota relates the following dream (diurnal residues are related to Gabriela having a cold and Carlota running into her neighbour, with whom she had a quarrel when she first moved to the building):

> I was in my bed feeling very tired, wanting to sleep and very sleepy and Daniela and Gabriela were there; suddenly the neighbour arrives and tells me that we have to get out of the house, that there is a war, I look through my window and I see collapsed buildings, rubble, a great disaster; I say to myself how could I have fallen asleep and not been aware of this.

Carlota starts crying inconsolably; she tells me, "I blame myself for not been more careful while I was pregnant with Andrea and for taking the prescribed drug." Carlota continues with her dream:

> I get out of bed and I realise that I am not wearing any clothes, no shoes, and that I can't leave with nothing on. I start looking for my clothes and suddenly a group of hired assassins (linked to a Mexican drug cartel), a group of very evil people, arrives and tells me that they are going to punish everybody who has high purchasing power, everybody who lives in places like my apartment. I realise that I am unable to escape but I ask them, crying, begging, to let my youngest daughter go to her grandmother's house, she is so young, to please let my girl go. Suddenly, and in another scene, her husband Alberto arrives and tells her, "I know how we can escape. Over there is a space through which we can get to our apartment (he means the previous apartment, but in the dream it is the same one); but be careful with that man, he wants to hurt you, do not go where he says. He is disobeying the rules, it is a group of evil people who follow some rules to do justice, but he does not." In the meantime, I see myself trying to convince a woman who is at the bottom of the group's hierarchy, but it seems that she is kind and will help us to escape; she is undecided, and suddenly the group's leader arrives and asks the woman why she is doing that and says that he is going to kill her.

Carlota observes how he takes out a gun, loads it, puts it to Carlota's temple, and suddenly she screams and wakes up.

Carlota associates the desolate place that was left in ruins with her family's current situation, her home after Andrea's death, knocked down. She associates her husband's wish to go back in time, to return to the old apartment where she became pregnant with Andrea (they moved out of the old apartment just three or four months before the birth because they needed a larger one). Their wish to escape with their two girls from the terrible tragedy in which they still are immersed is evident. Carlota associates that her gynaecologist "is the evil man from my dream, who is now telling me that I did not leave the hospital immediately, and that he did not prescribe the drug." As a first approximation, I interpret that perhaps a part of her is like this group that, despite being evil, are seeking justice, the part of her that feels evil because she could not protect Andrea and for that reason she thinks she deserves a punishment. The other part of her is the one that was paralysed because of the sorrow and pain, and without finding a way out, she is still trapped in her suffering, with nothing to protect her. Likewise, there is still aggression inside her. We continue working with the dream's multiple meanings and with her recovery process, assimilation, and self-forgiveness, and she says goodbye again.

Discussion

Carlota developed a maternal transference towards me, she perceived me as "the good mother" who could support her and ease her pain, who understood her suffering; she felt supported by me, she knew that she could call me any time; she felt my empathy, and the trust that came from having a successful previous treatment. Also, my recommendation of her husband's therapy and her daughter's, and later couple therapy, all ended successfully.

A key aspect of Carlota's treatment was related to the countertransference, since, as an analyst and grandmother, I had recently gone through a very similar event that resulted in the death of my new-born grandson. I mention here the deep empathy derived from the resonances that Carlota's discourse had on me, when I was thoroughly convinced of the health professionals' negligence in both events. It is important to note that her unspeakable pain, suffering, and affliction, were mine as well, of both families.

Regarding the technique used, in the first stage of treatment a weekly session of psychoanalytic psychotherapy was provided for fourteen consecutive months (about fifty-six sessions). From the neonatal death onwards, an intervention model that integrated two therapeutic modalities was provided: the first one was the multimodal psychotherapy for families at high psychosocial risk (Maldonado Durán & Lartigue, 2002) and the second was Winnicott's (1971, 1989) on demand treatment, complemented by Lebovici (1983) and Solís Pontón (2002; Solís Pontón et al., 2006).

It is important that psychoanalysts and psychotherapists who provide care to bereaved families consider the contributions of those authors who have furthered the psychodynamic understanding of perinatal loss. Of note are the works of Leon (1986, 1987, 1990, 1992, 1996), Mazet and Lebovici (1996), and Raphael-Leff (2011). In addition, the work of Aray (1967) and Pines (1990), related to abortion, and the work of Bleichmar (2010), related to pathological mourning, the grieving stages described by Kubler-Ross (1968), and Kohner and Henley's (1995) principles of good practice.

The treatment of bereaved families after neonatal death involves learning to cope with the only irreparable thing that is dead, where anything that is done will not modify the loss of the child: a loss that can destroy the psychological functioning of the parents and the family structure (nuclear and extended family), especially when there is no self-forgiveness. Vives (2013) asks what are the dynamics of the mental apparatus that promote the superego being able to forgive the ego for an irreparable event in the reality of the external world, signified in the fantasy of the internal world? Although he states that there is still no answer to this question, he suggests that

> Some evolutionary late components of the censoring instance include some capacity for judgement and love for the ego, and we therefore believe that the superego is not only fuelled by the death wish, but also contains important libidinal components. It is possible that the dynamics of internal forgiveness are related to some form of equilibrium of forces, in the core of the superego, between the mortiferous forces and the distinctive elements of life and love. (p. 176, translated for this edition)

Surviving a tragic experience with all the responsibility that this implies is not an easy task for families who face the painful and terrible loss of a child and, without doubt, this has a fundamental emotional impact on their existences (Vives, 2013).

Acknowledgement

The author gratefully acknowledges the assistance of Dr José Cuenca in the preparation of the English translation.

References

Aray, J. (1967). *Aborto: Un Estudio Psicoanalítico*. Buenos Aires: Paidós.

Bleichmar, H. (2010). Rethinking pathological mourning: multiple types and therapeutic approaches. *Psychoanalytic Quarterly, 79*: 71–93.

Cain, A. C., & Cain, B. S. (1964). On replacing a child. *Journal of the American Academy of Child & Adolescent Psychiatry, 3*: 443–455.

Kohner, N., & Henley, A. (1995). *When a Baby Dies*. London: Harper Collins.

Kubler-Ross, E. (1968). *On Death and Dying*. New York: Macmillan.

Lanza-Castelli, G. (2010). Poner en palabras, mentalización y psicoterapia. *Aperturas Psicoanalíticas, 36*.

Lartigue, T. (2005). Los padres frente a las pérdidas perinatales. In: E. Dallal (Ed.), *Caminos del Desarrollo Psicológico: La Muerte* (pp. 195–221). México City: Plaza y Valdés,

Lartigue, T., & Maldonado-Durán, M. (1998). El síndrome del niño(a) de reemplazo: vicisitudes del desarrollo. In: T. Lartigue, M. Maldonado-Durán, & H. Avila Rosas (Eds.), *La Alimentación en la Primera Infancia y sus Efectos en el Desarrollo* (pp. 301–318). México City: Asociación Psicoanalítica Mexicana and Plaza y Valdés.

Lartigue, T., & Vives, J. (1994). Aspectos psicodinámicos del aborto espontáneo. In: S. Peña & M. Lemlij (Eds.), *Feminidad y Masculinidad: XX Congreso Latinoamericano de Psicoanálisis* (pp. 419–429). Lima: FEPAL.

Lebovici, S. (1983). *Le Nourrisson, la Mère et le Psychanalyste: Les Interactions Précoces*. Avec la coll. de S. Stoléru, Paris: Le Centurion.

Leon, I. (1986). Psychodynamics of perinatal loss. *Psychiatry, 49*: 312–324.

Leon, I. (1987). Short-term psychotherapy for perinatal loss. *Psychotherapy, 24*: 186–195.

Leon, I. (1990). *When a Baby Dies: Psychotherapy for Pregnancy and Newborn Loss*. New Haven, CT: Yale University Press.

Leon, I. (1992). The psychoanalytic conceptualisation of perinatal loss: a multi-dimensional model. *American Journal of Psychiatry, 149*: 1464–1472.

Leon, I. (1996). Revising psychoanalytic understandings of perinatal loss. *Psychoanalytic Psychology, 13*: 161–176.

López, R., Lartigue, T., González, G., & de la Cerda, D. (1997). Descripción de una intervención psicodinámica con embarazo del alto riesgo y experiencia de pérdida perinatal. *Revista Mexicana de Psicología, 14*: 65–74.

Losso, R. (2001). *Psicoanálisis de la Familia: Recorridos Teórico-Clínicos*. Buenos Aires: Lumen.

Maldonado-Duran, J. M., & Lartigue, T. (2002). Multimodal parent–infant psychotherapy. In: J. M. Maldonado-Durán (Ed.), *Infant and Toddler Mental Health: Models of Clinical Intervention* (pp. 129–160). Washington, DC: American Psychiatric Press.

Maldonado-Durán, M., Morales-Monsalve, M., Gómez, K., Maher, A., Brown, M., & Camacho-Durán, A. (2013). Consecuencias de los eventos traumáticos sufridos por la madre en la relación con sus hijos. Paper presented to the 48th International Congress of the International Psychoanalytical Association, Prague, July.

Mazet, P., & Lebovici, S. (1996). *Mort Subite du Nourrisson: Un Deuil Impossible?* Paris: Presses Universitaires de France.

Pines, D. (1990). Pregnancy, miscarriage and abortion. *International Journal of Psychoanalysis, 71*: 301–307.

Raphael-Leff, J. (2011). *Spilt Milk: Perinatal Loss and Breakdown*. London: Karnac.

Solís Pontón, L. (2002). *La Parentalidad, Desafío para el Tercer Milenio: Un Homenaje Internacional a Serge Lebovici*. México City: Manual Moderno.

Solís Pontón, L., Lartigue, T., & Maldonado Durán, M. (2006). *La Cultura de la Parentalidad: Antídoto Contra la Violencia y la Barbarie*. México City: Manual Moderno.

Vives, J. (2013). *Lo Irreparable y Otros Ensayos Psicoanalíticos*. México City: Editores de Textos Mexicanos.

Vives, J., & Lartigue, T. (2003). De la pareja a la familia. In: E. Dallal (Ed.), *Caminos del Desarrollo Psicológico: De la Edad Adulta a la Vejez* (pp. 149–199). México City: Plaza y Valdés.

Winnicott, D. W. (1971). Therapeutic consultations in child psychiatry. London: Hogarth Press.

Winnicott, D. W. (1989). *Psicoanálisis de una Niña Pequeña* [The Piggle: An Account of the Psychoanalytic Treatment of a Little Girl]. Buenos Aires: Gedisa.

CHAPTER SIX

Adolescent maternity in critical social context: a perspective from the psychoanalyst's *hilflosigkeit*

Ema Ponce de León Leiras

Introduction

The issue of adolescent maternity requires that we reconsider our ideas on adolescence in view of the proposal of several authors who prefer to talk about "adolescences". This emerges from evidence that the socio-cultural context leads to new clinical interventions that will work within the framework of subjectivity and the social aspects that run through it. Our theories and concepts remain an essential reference, but should be more open than ever to question and transformation, just like the analyst's mind itself.

My experience in this subject arises from my work as a psychotherapist in Casa Lunas, a non-government organisation (NGO) (www.casalunas.org) in Montevideo dedicated to the care of adolescent mothers in a precarious social position with their children and partners.

First, I would like to emphasise that *maternity and adolescence have a unique subjective dimension and, at the same time, are social constructs*, thus, the specificity of adolescent maternity relates to the socio-cultural determinants of each particular period, region, and social stratum.

Social perspective and intervention positioning in the face of adolescent maternity

Throughout history, most women have become mothers while in the age group that is today called "adolescence". According to the World Health Organization (WHO), it is the period between childhood and adulthood that ranges from ten to twenty years of age. Therefore, this is not a new phenomenon. The social and economic changes of the twentieth century, which include the term "adolescence", give us a new perspective on maternity at this stage of life.

What happens today with adolescent maternity? The WHO (2014) reports that eleven per cent of babies worldwide are born to mothers aged between fifteen and nineteen. Ninety-five per cent of these births occur in low- and middle-income countries.

In our clinical work in general, but especially with phenomena that contradict what a given society considers appropriate, it becomes important to understand and deconstruct the ideological and cultural determinants and the myths contained in the social imaginary, either the imaginary on its own, or of the individuals it intends to help.

We should keep in mind that maternity is a complex and multivocal phenomenon. Throughout history and across cultures, it has changed in its practices and in the social imaginary. The individuals of different times, different cultures, and different social segments are the spokespeople of conflicts between current socio-cultural mandates and what emerges from the individual's background, the underlying transgenerational sediment, not only at a family level, but also at a social level.

These conflicts express the tension between current and past cultural elements. What is the value of maternity in society? What is the role of the father in the family structure? How do maternal and paternal functions interrelate? Is maternity a social mandate or a choice? What are the roles of institutions, society, and the state with regard to maternity, etc.?

We must not lose sight of the strong ideological aspect that affects our positions depending on the culture in which we are immersed. We always confront what is different, and we must leave aside our professional knowledge to "learn" about an unknown and complex reality and, from there, design ways to intervene.

In the socio-cultural context of a globalised world, in which middle-class women have accessed education and employment almost equally to men, and maternity appears as an option, *adolescent maternity is identified as a problem to be avoided*. This is supported in specific discourses of academic literature that highlight a focus on risk from a medical, social, and psychological point of view. However, in today's societies with severe social and economic crises, this phenomenon should be questioned beyond our preconceptions.

Pereira (2012) states: "The hegemonic visions in society are usually constructed by adults . . . the institutions tend to reproduce an adult-centred culture that reinforces the passive and subordinate place of adolescents in society" (p. 101).

With this vision in mind, other authors emphasise the importance of not reinforcing the idea that a child is an obstacle to the achievement of other social objectives, revaluing the experience of parenthood (Wilson & Huntington, 2005). Likewise, Duncan (2007) suggests that, rather than crystallisation and confirmation of the specific situation of exclusion, it can be taken as an opportunity out of this situation, if the potential that can be developed is taken into account.

We, therefore, propose a situational focus. This means that every situation is unique and must be considered that way. We cannot anticipate that adolescent maternity will have negative consequences, not to mention the increased vulnerability of overcoming two critical processes simultaneously. As Vives and Lartigue de Vives (1991) say, the normal crisis of pregnancy overlaps with the normal crisis of adolescence, struggling with biological and psychological processes of both. We think that there is greater risk when, in addition to these factors, there is also a situation of poverty and social exclusion before the pregnancy.

While in Western societies today we see that in the middle and upper-middle classes the onset of maternity is postponed due to women taking on jobs, in classes with fewer resources, the onset of maternity is at an earlier age. For young girls from the poorest sectors of society, with difficulties in entering and remaining in the educational system and accessing the labour market, maternity is seen as a way to socially integrate through a valued role, rushing headlong into the adult world but without the resources for sustainability.

The situational focus allows for the inclusion of the subjective perspective that relates to the experiences and unique circumstances of each case, offering devices that take into account the peculiarities of this population, depending on the stage of life they are in, but, at the same time, with a social perspective that addresses the social problems that are the major risk factor for the future. It is, therefore, about the answers that include the subject–society dialectic.

Psychoanalytic views of adolescence today and adolescent maternity in vulnerable social contexts

The work of the psychoanalyst in institutions and communities gives rise to the real challenge we face in the twenty-first century: the opportunity to create and develop clinical interventions that enable a real interface between psychoanalysis and the demands of social reality. It not only requires a different positioning from the psychoanalyst from that of the consulting room, without giving up their identity, in a new transformative twist. They must tolerate a place of greater vulnerability and uncertainty as to the external and internal variables in line with the context in which they are immersed.

We will consider some aspects of adolescence in the light of the social context in which we develop our work with adolescent mothers. It is a context with economic problems, emotional deprivation, absence or instability of family ties, and where violence and abandonment are common. In these cases, adolescent transition is marked by the effects of a cumulative traumatic component often originating in the early stages, and lasting through childhood until adolescence. It has a strong imprint of the social conditions that add to the historical uniqueness. Therefore, these individuals have more psychological vulnerability and few elements of environmental support to face the changes and the new internal and external requirements of this stage of life. At the same time, we also note the presence of unique resources assisting in the mental survival and adaptation to the reality in which they live.

The common denominator of *hilflosigkeit* (helplessness) results in a greater urgency to meet all kinds of demands, as well as transgressions, in order to obtain what they want fast. This is often channelled through drug use. The omnipotent child, who has not been able to develop in an appropriate framework of dependence, is present in full force, resisting the feelings of growing up.

We understand that the different challenges faced by adolescents are intensified, or especially hampered, in youth in precarious or marginal social contexts. We propose reviewing some of them, following the lines of a recent publication by a Uruguayan colleague on psychoanalysis and adolescence (Casas, 2011), who highlights vulnerability as the common denominator in all-time adolescence. We summarise aspects that this author develops and which we believe are central to the way we understand the adolescent process. This is a stage where there is an attempt at social repositioning of men and women, the redefinition of identities, resorting to peer groups to deny or hate whatever is different, thus leading to discrimination. Redefinition not only involves oedipal, but also narcissistic, levels. That is to say, not only is it a question of taking hold of the parental and social other, but also achieving discrimination and a limit to the other's knowledge through hate and aggressiveness. Hence, the importance of recognition and generational care, as opposed to indifference towards the object which causes deep narcissistic injuries. Resorting to omnipotence to confront the limits and experiences of helplessness and fragility is frequent. The act is an essential part of the adolescent discourse, as well as actions.

García (2011) highlights two markers of subjective appropriation that occur in adolescence: the generational rupture required for subjectivity and the appropriation of the adult body and the exercise of sexuality, always in conflict, reminding one that sexual initiation is a source of distress facing the unknown.

For our part, we would add the urgency of the drive, the central place of the body as an axis of transformation, the pivot of what is shown in acts and messages to be decoded, vehicles of meaning that we will try to integrate into thinking. In many cases, pregnancy can be conceived of as an enactment, or also as a performance, a way out from a conflicted internal situation, whether or not it involves a repetition linked to individual or family history. It can give substance to aspects of idealisation, a way to hold on to the illusory, faced with an intolerable reality. We can also notice a rush into an adult role in the face of the fragility of identification figures. It is about paternity or maternity providing a stronger masculine or feminine identity, taking hold of the other through a role, of some traits, while entertaining a simultaneous illusion of differentiating themselves: "I will be a father or mother different to the one I had". However, we know how difficult it is to escape repetition, despite the reparative processes that are set in motion, which are successful in many cases. In this respect, "Maternity and paternity sometimes operate as a driving force for the acquisition of new means of orientation for life" (Beech, 2012, p. 14).

As to the processes of resignifying identification, there is a distinctive complexity in adolescents who become pregnant. We have observed the search for recreation of the maternal relationship, whether in a fusional movement through regressive identification with the infant, or otherwise in a negative Oedipus movement, giving the mother the baby to care for as if the baby were part of herself that she is afraid of growing up, a typical paradox of adolescence, since, at the same time, she also becomes a mother. Another course is the need to complete or repair failed processes of identification with an absent or abandoning identificatory figure.

Regarding the body and the mobilisation of body image that occurs in adolescence, pregnancy adds a major transformation that impacts differently according to the prevailing ghosts and pregenital and phallic records at stake. The "belly" can embody fantasies of phallic completeness that belie castration, or incestuous fantasies through bodily deformation, experienced with shame, since they reveal a sexual transgression. Although these ghosts do not differ from those that pregnancy can summon in an adult woman, these are closer to childhood roots in a period of restructuring movements and, therefore, they can happen with greater harshness and intensity.

Depending on the psychological resources in each case, these ghosts and the ever-present ambivalence can be developed and distinguished from actual pregnancy, influenced by the perception of the baby as a separate individual and the narcissistic libidinal contribution generated, as well as the affection awakened.

This means that in full adolescent urges and narcissistic commotion, maternity cannot but play a significant role in how the psychological restructuring at stake is approached. Pregnancy shows a transformed body, enlarged and marked by the presence of a child to be born and a form of appropriation of genital sexuality. Even though it is not in itself a sign of sexual maturation, through actions, sexuality shows its effects on the body as in no other way. Showing the body as source of life can assist in the affirmation against experiences of psychological destruction linked to death, violence, lack of affection, and abandonment.

According to Peña and Buchwald (2011), some phenomena stand out as common in the clinical work with pregnant adolescents.

1. Failure in the separation–individuation process of the mother herself: through the child, they relive unity and, at the same time, the impossibility of separating.
2. A deficit in narcissism in times of early construction of the psychological apparatus, where the child and/or partner restore the lost unity through "being-with the other".
3. A search to verify fertility and an imaginary completeness through pregnancy, with the crisis coming with the birth and upbringing of the child

Non-resolution of these conflicts gives rise to regressive episodes, where the child is experienced as a sibling with whom they compete for maternal care and where they fail to separate from their families of origin. However, there are adolescents who achieve a level of new maturity by incorporating the maternal role as part of their identity.

Thus, paradoxical situations arise in several respects. The subjective motivations of those who become pregnant in their teens are often related to the search for certain narcissistic balances already mentioned above, which, for that unique life circumstance, may be the best alternative for psychological homeostasis. We must not forget that these pregnancies frequently raise the question of abortion, and the conscious or unconscious choice has been to continue pregnancy. That is, without disregarding the unfavourable social conditions, we must consider the role occupied by desire and the attempt at change and assuming an active position that are at stake. Therefore, institutions must deal with a complex mesh of variables, aiming to make nascent parenting an opportunity for social inclusion and that it be positively integrated in the construction of the identity process.

What can the psychoanalyst contribute in the framework of an institution?

Ponce de León & Schroeder (2011) suggest that

> As psychoanalysts we can make specific contributions to the social and symbolic dimensions of exclusion, in the framework of organisations,

> teams and institutions, both with our individual or group therapeutic approach and through *the care of the caregiver*, promoting in all cases permanent construction of subjectivity and social bonds. (Translated for this edition)

With regard to the care of the carer, psychoanalysts who have group training can perform a relevant role within teams that work with social problems. Schroeder (2008) points out:

> The manifest work of such groups is hampered by the latencies at stake: excess of violence, abused sexualities, bare impulses, unthinkable abandonments. Nobody comes out unscathed when, together with others, they seek to promote inclusion processes, "recycling" processes from which they have been previously "left out" in the margins of our societies . . . [It is about] promoting elaboration processes, working the resistances and obstacles that appear in the work, noticing the blind spots, possible "acting" or omnipotent attitudes, as well as feelings of helplessness, falling into inactivity and depression. (p. 149, translated for this edition)

Hence, the importance of creating group mechanisms for reflection within institutions.

I agree with Viñar (2009) that "work with marginalised groups and extreme traumatic situations" is the experience that most clearly shows us the

> biased and restrictive nature of a clinical approach that only . . . emphasises . . . unconscious causation as determinant of the psychological structuring and leads us to explore other territories and other conceptual itineraries. (p. 88)

As to my personal experience in this field, I have mainly participated as a psychoanalyst in Casa Lunas, and I believe that individual care cannot be separated from the therapeutic effects of the institutional environment. In a time of high psychological permeability such as adolescence, it enables a process of restructuring identifications in providing an environment that we could describe, in Winnicott's terms, as facilitating and supportive. The ties with professionals are formed in a space and atmosphere that is, at the same time, familiar and exogamous, at times with the role of a protecting family and at others of a differentiated social environment that favours autonomy.

The experience is sufficiently long and continued as to leave a strong imprint in adolescents who commit to it, a place where a story and subjectivity are constructed.

Life stories: Marcelo and Mabela

Marcelo and Mabela, fifteen and sixteen years old, respectively, met at a juvenile care institution and then lived on the streets, where they conceived Eva. I got in touch with them at a postpartum workshop. They were living then in a room in Marcelo's father's house; he was an alcoholic, who was physically violent to his son. Marcelo has a domineering and possessive attitude towards Mabela, who disappears in his presence and talks very little, in contrast to his poise. They established a fusional link between each other that, at the same time, is violent, with episodes in which Marcelo hits her and, on one occasion, he slapped the baby when she was almost one year old. On these occasions, Mabela has asked for help and they sometimes separated, but for just a few days. Mabela always returns and he despairs in her absence.

At the workshop, Marcelo stated,

> I had been waiting since I was twelve to have a child. I met Mabela and we sought to have a baby together. Everything changes, the way of thinking, of seeing life. I stopped using drugs for my daughter. I learnt more on the streets than from society. If you are discriminated against, you don't exist. Grandparents change, now I get along better with my mother, it is different since I have my daughter.

Marcelo is one of the few fathers who attend the centre daily. In it, he plays a very active role, participating in several workshops and artisanal ventures. He likes being the only male in the group and feels threatened when other fathers show up. This is connected with the desire for a daughter. He seeks to be liked, to conquer the affection of the personnel and young mothers. He is very impulsive and is under psychiatric treatment, but does not accept psychotherapy. He has had episodes of transgression, stealing in Casa Lunas, but has only been suspended, not expelled.

The conflicted relationship of the couple raises concerns in the institution. Mabela is offered individual psychotherapy with me, which she readily accepts, attending regularly. Psychotherapy is conducted with her and the baby. In contrast to her silent role in the group, Mabela talks non-stop. She lost her mother when she was one and then her father; both died of AIDS. She tells a story marked by criminal and violent acts. At the age of seven, she was raped by her grandmother's partner. She describes multiple episodes populated by characters who rapidly enter and leave the scene, showing the spatial–temporal confusion of her life and her psyche. I perceive the value she attaches to the transmission of that complex genealogy made up of the missing, the imprisoned, rapists, murderers, and murder victims. She shows me that she has survived all possible extreme situations. She says proudly,

> Who would remember all this? I do. When someone insults my mother I defend her, you see her picture and we are identical. I want to be a hairdresser, because all women in my family trained as hairdressers. Eva is like me when I was a baby. I love her a lot because I don't have my mum. She didn't take care of herself, but I will take care of myself because of my daughter, so that the same thing doesn't happen to her.

She shows no anguish when describing situations in which she was subjected to violence. Substantial depressive aspects are evident in her lack of hygiene and personal care. While I listen to and watch her, I feel moved by the quality of her relationship with the baby, with whom she has found moments of happiness unknown to her. The naturalness of her maternal gestures contrasts with her verbose account, the intertwining of multiple discourses, myths, and stories put together by all the "others" in her short but intense life: relatives, neighbours, and institutions. Later on, she will tell us, "I took out what was inside me, it was a relief for me, I had never spoken of my things in this way . . ."

In the course of her treatment over nearly a year, there are episodes of jealousy by Marcelo towards her, infidelity on his part, separations and reconciliations, which meant working with experiences of helplessness, extreme dependence, and violence between them. Marcelo's aggressiveness seems to be a protective feature against external violence and Mabela's difficulty in acknowledging her desires and setting limits. While in other cases it is necessary to work through difficulties with the maternal role, this is not the case with Mabela.

In one of their separations, Mabela leaves Marcelo because he is again heavily using drugs. She tells me that he looked for her in the streets, and when she went to collect the welfare payment for the baby, he stole the money from her. Very hurt and furious with what had happened, she reported him to the police. She says that she felt very bad and that she could not understand how he could steal his daughter's money: "If I had parents this wouldn't happen." It is very hard for her to think, and she transmits a kind of mental vacuum to me, where she can only talk about facts and acts. It does not seem that she can hear me, except for indicating her "total disillusionment" and her desire to take revenge on Marcelo.

Mabela is placed with her daughter in a carer's house, but before long she absconds with another adolescent mother. Abandoning different INAU (Institute for Children and Adolescents of Uruguay) homes to live on the streets has been a constant in her past. This time, after fifteen days, she gives her daughter to her brother and sister-in-law, a place where Mabela knows Eva will be well cared for.

Therapeutic work is suspended. The institution serves as a meeting place, twice a week, between Mabela and Eva. According to the information I receive, the encounters between them are good, affectionate, and moments of separation are emotional but adequate. I came across her on one of those days and I offered to meet her whenever she requested to do so. Her request reaches me immediately.

Mabela has grown worse; she is gaunt, with new clothes, but with a strong odour due to lack of hygiene. She looks older. She tells me that she is smoking a lot of marijuana to forget all about her daughter. She sleeps in the open with a new partner who is a user. I listen to her story, consisting mainly of facts. My intervention is centred on recounting the narrative of her return to the streets after the episode where Marcelo stole the money from her, destroying her trust and confidence. I point out to her that she tolerated being beaten by him, but his stealing meant that he did not love her or his daughter, that nothing was worth anything, that nothing mattered. She feels like discarded litter, a piece of shit, and, therefore, the place for her to be is on the streets, where Marcelo stole from her. She nods as tears roll down her face. While crying, she tells me that when she goes to visit Eva at her brother's house, Eva tells her, "I love you" and caresses her face. These words to describe the pain of loss and abandonment, of being subject to violence and disaffection, and to give up and let go of everything do not come near to expressing the significance of the situation.

I propose to resume our weekly work to try to understand what happens to her and why she does not want to be in an INAU home and accept the support offered to her, knowing that in order to be with her daughter she has to leave the streets. The reason she can state most clearly refers to freedom to do what she wants, to having no restrictions on her desires, to the fact that there she could not have her mobile phone at her disposal. We hold some meetings until she leaves the institution, which coincides with the end of the year.

From hilflosigkeit *to the hope of the therapeutic bond*

We want to transmit two lines of reflection emerging from the oscillation of the analyst's feelings between moments of powerlessness and helplessness and those of hope and confidence that patients unexpectedly give us.

Subjectivation and parenthood in social helplessness

How can the processes of subjectivation and parenthood in these young people be considered where historical trauma is cumulative and multiple, leading to cycles of repetition of violence and helplessness? To understand the difficulties with parenthood, prevalent in the midst of highly deprivation, the concept of "affiliation", defined by Gutton (2006) is useful:

> The psychological elaboration of an individual . . . to acquire, possess what they inherited from fathers and mothers, whereby the individual integrates, reproduces, reconstructs, and restores in the *après coup* the legacies of the raw transmission in order to make it into a serviceable object without which it would remain . . . not able to be represented with the rest of the psychic life. (p. 21, translated for this edition)

Effort in the affiliation process is clearly expressed by Mabela at the beginning of her treatment. A great difficulty in the possibility of subjectivation is that of having to carry out the mental work of affiliation, which is essentially symbolic, based on a transgenerational chain with multiple abrupt cessations, violations of the law, and of incest, an accumulation of horrors and fragments that cannot be represented. The paradox lies in that the genuine transmission material, which has to be integrated as part of the person's own story, is, in itself, full of symbolic ruptures.

A major difficulty is added when, in the midst of this laborious process of identity construction, in their passage through maternity and paternity, repetition of violence and transgressive effects occur, which attack those incipient functions. These repetitions involve the individual story but also that which is transgenerational and the current social dimension. This occurs when Marcelo steals Eva's welfare payment from Mabela. With that act, Marcelo destroys the possibility of ownership of a paternal function in both of them. What was being precariously constructed in Mabela collapses with the repetition of another who abandons, attacks and breaches essential codes. Mabela does not tolerate living alone with her daughter at an institution; she prefers living on the streets again. She gives her daughter to her brother, as representative of her parentage, in a transaction between the endogamic and an attempt to rescue some trait of paternal function, leaving us with multiple questions about the vicissitudes of parenthood and the psychological scars in these adolescents.

Mabela asked herself something like: who can survive all this, all that I have experienced, when faced with a feeling of failure of the constancy of object love, as much of being invested in as investing in the other, the boundlessly open space on the streets, having nowhere to turn, having nothing, and with no possibilities? Being on the streets might represent the opposite to affiliation, an immeasurable open space of anonymity, full of objects that challenge and enact the urges before the void and rupture of affiliation ties, a space of omnipotent control and indiscriminate approval, both everybody's and no-mans-land. Exclusive ownership of some does not exist there, and appropriation of what is not their own may be exercised almost as a right.

Finally, we ask ourselves if seeking pregnancy and a child are not, in these contexts, something we already pointed out, a way of making sexual aspects and life predominate over violence and death, and of promoting the linkage of the erotic and the thanatic, the latter inherent in the acted violence so prevalent in excluded social sectors. In these situations, we observe how the offer of an intimate space, of availability and committed listening, might mean an opportunity to repair "something" in a fabric full of holes and broken threads. However, it is just a small link in a chain of resources that always fall short of repairing the extreme damage already inflicted on the social fabric.

These speculations are part of the effort to translate into known concepts what escapes us and a subject who gets lost to us because of constraints, or our own socio-cultural aspect. The challenge ahead is, in any case, to persist, develop theoretical concepts and psychoanalytic practices which occur as an effect of the face-to-face encounter, in the inherent helplessness of the analyst confronting these issues.

Meeting Mabela again: a shoot of life

A year and a half after our last encounter, and coinciding with my writing of the previous reflections in this chapter, Mabela lets me know through the NGO of her desire to meet with me. This deeply moved me.

Sitting at a table, Mabela's first gesture is her extended hand looking for mine. We are both moved. She has come because she is worried about Eva, the fact that she is seeing her less because of restrictions on her brother's part because of some attempts by her to take the child without authorisation. Mabela tells me about many things that occurred in this period. She lives with a much older man, whom she says treats her well; she has a roof and food and feels well cared for. She wants me to help her talk with her brother because she does not have the courage. I tell her that she finds it difficult to make herself heard and respected by men, as used to happen with Marcelo.

The central topic in our encounters was imagining a future that enables her to keep close to her daughter, and the importance for her to work, doing anything, since she does nothing the whole day except watching television or sleeping. We see each other about four times, interspersed with some absences, where I keep waiting for her and she does not come. The institution makes the last communication between us possible, which is made by telephone. She is happy; for the past two months she has been working in a restaurant kitchen at night and tells me that is the reason she failed to come to our last meetings, as she fell asleep. She tells me that because she is working her brother respects her in a different way and allows her to see Eva again. This re-encounter with Mabela shows that, even in extreme cases, repetition is not alike each time and that small and large steps of transformation from what happened before are possible: small if we consider our ideal, large if we put ourselves in the shoes of Mabela.

Mabela made her voice heard to find me; she could communicate her anguish to me, listen to what arose from our exchange, and modify her situation in relation to what she understood. If we look at her current life, not from our preconceptions but in relation to what she experienced before, she is no longer living on the streets or with an abuser, as all her previous partners were, but with someone who takes care of her. For the first time in her life, she succeeds in getting a job and receiving a salary.

Considering it from a parenting model in which the mother lives together with her children and provides care daily, we could say that she has given up her maternal role. But why not consider it from other possible models, when aspects that also have to do with the maternal may be preserved? Mabela did not abandon Eva, she is not exposing her to life on the streets, she takes care of her more than she takes care of herself, putting her in the hands of her brother and his partner, in a family structure that gives her affection and the material care and stability she cannot give her herself.

She continues to exercise her maternal role as much as she can. They spend weekends together, she starts work driven by her love of her daughter and her desire not to lose the bond that she is building from a different place, which is not the repetition of her own story. We may formulate the idea, following Winnicott's line of thought, that "good enough" motherhood is one that develops itself creatively in order to adapt to the real and internal possibilities of each individual in their different life circumstances.

There are surely other stories and other Mabelas to teach us to take a fresh look at that which, from our ideals and preconceptions, could be another link in the transgenerational chain of failed and traumatic maternities and paternities. However, we could also consider the possibility of an identifying redefinition, in which the abandonment that marks their primary ties could, to some extent, be transformed.

We believe this was possible thanks to the support, continuity, and trust provided by the tie with the NGO during her daughter's first eighteen months, and the therapeutic tie, which were both simultaneous and harmonious. Mabela shows us that it is possible to build ties that are different to the past, and that a therapeutic encounter, in which a symbolising container may be co-created, is not as futile as we might sometimes believe. Paths are created and some seeds silently wait until they can see the light. It does not matter how small the shoot is or how much it will grow, it is about life.

References

Beech, J. (2012). Foreword. In: A. Pergalli A. & J. Sampietro (Eds.), *Maternidades, paternidades y adolescencias* (pp. 11–15). Buenos Aires: Noveduc Libros.

Casas, M. (2011). Adolescencia. In: S. Flechner (Ed.), *Psicoanálisis y Adolescencia. Dos temporalidades que se interpelan* (pp. 19–43). Montevideo: Psicolibros.

Duncan, S. (2007). "What's the problem with teenage parents? And what's the problem with the policy? *Critical Social Policy, 27*: 307–328.

García, S. (2011). Adolescencia, violencia y subjetivación. In: S. Flechner (Ed.), *Psicoanálisis y Adolescencia* (pp. 85–93). Montevideo: Psicolibros.

Gutton, Ph. (2006). GREUPP. *Adolescence, 55*(1): 9–32.

Peña, M., & Buchwald, M. (2011). La maternidad en la adolescencia. Su dimensión subjetiva. In: *Travesías del cuerpo femenino. Un recorrido Psicoanalítico en torno a temas de Ginecología y Obstetricia* (pp. 105–120). Buenos Aires: Letra Viva.

Pereira, J. (2012). Academia, política e instituciones, problemas en las miradas adultas sobre la maternidad y la paternidad en la adolescencia. In: A. Pergalli & J. Sampietro (Eds.), *Maternidades, paternidades y adolescencias* (pp. 101–122). Buenos Aires: Noveduc Libros.

Ponce de León, E., & Schroeder, D. (2011). Maternité adolescente dans des contextes d'exclusion et globalisation. Paper presented to the Congrès des cinq Continents, Lyon, 19–22 October.

Schroeder, D. (2008). Exclusión social. Aportes del psicoanálisis a los procesos de inclusión. In*: Exclusión–Inclusión. II Coloquio Emergencia social. Asociación Psicoanalítica del Uruguay* (*Volumen VIII*) (pp. 144–151). Montevideo: Biblioteca Uruguaya de Psicoanálisis.

Viñar, M. (2009). *Mundos Adolescentes y vértigo civilizatorio*. Montevideo: Ediciones Trilce.

Vives, J., & Lartigue de Vives, T. (1991). Viscisitudes de la identidad femenina en la maternidad precoz. *Revista de Psicoanálisis, XLVIII*(4): 767–776.

Wilson, H., & Huntington, A. (2005). Deviant mothers: the construction of teenage motherhood in contemporary discourse. *Journal of Social Policy, 35*(1): 59–76.

World Health Organization (WHO) (2014). Adolescent pregnancy: www.who.int/mediacentre/factsheets/fs364/en/

PART II

NEW FAMILY CONFIGURATIONS

CHAPTER SEVEN

Vicissitudes of the desire to have a child in contemporary parenthoods: reproductive techniques and the new origins

Patricia Alkolombre

Introduction

The place of the desire to have a child is the guiding thread and point of departure of this chapter. It is a central issue in parenthood, especially when techniques of assisted fertilisation are used. It is linked, on the one hand, to parental desires and, on the other hand, to the child's identity in relation to knowledge of the child's origins.

These are current topics of interest, and, therefore, the participation of psychoanalysis in these debates is quite important. It is no less important that we enquire into what is permanent in comparison to what is changing in these scenarios, based on clinical observation.

The vicissitudes of the desire to have a child in contemporary parenthoods lead us to think about and explore their scope in psychoanalytic clinical work. Technology has introduced a new order in procreation, in the manner of an event (Badiou, 1988), leading, in turn, to new ways of filiation.

Contemporary maternities and paternities

Parenthoods are no longer what they were, and this process is irreversible. We all know that the traditional ways of being conceived—in the intimacy of a sexual relation—are many thousands of years old, whereas those initiated with medical–technological intervention began little more than thirty years ago.

They represent a change of paradigm in the mode of constitution of families, and their social and cultural context is specific. They started with the discovery of the contraceptive pill in the 1960s, which radically dissociated sexual activity from the arrival of children. Twenty years later, this equation was inverted with the implementation of assisted fertilisation techniques: it became possible to have children without having sexual relations.

Since then, culture has intervened with a new order in sexuality and procreation, influencing the vicissitudes of the desire to have a child in men and women. New forms of cohabitation between genders became possible, and power relations between men and women changed.

We recall the era of "free love" when, for the first time in the history of humanity, sexual life diverged radically from biological determinants of sexual desire by becoming independent of the period of fertility. Later, changes in the reproductive field arrived and the traditional ways of conceiving children became history.

At this time, very different ways of filiation share a context of sexual diversity, including single parenthoods and homo-parenthoods, both masculine and feminine. These transformations disturb symbolic references, in the words of Tort (1994). He concludes that these changes affect the structures of symbolic systems governing the identification of subjects in all known societies, such as filiation, maternity, paternity, and sexuated identity.

We are living in a unique historical period, a transition between generations born before the implementation of reproductive technologies, which we could name the "pre-test-tube" era, when men and women lived with natural fertility and adoption as the only possible ways to constitute families. In contrast, current generations are immersed in changes brought about by the use of contraceptives and assisted fertility, which have led to greater freedom and diversity in filiation projects. In this sense, we are privileged witnesses to explain this historical transition and explore its repercussions on subjectivity.

Kaës (2001) proposed that the introduction of a third, technical–medical element in reproduction radically modifies birth and its representations, and, thereby, acquires a tertiary position in fertility:

> This is done by three, and therefore the medical technique is involved as a fertilising and parental agency. We do not yet know what modifications are introduced in the relations between generations and the child's status. Neither do we know what effects these technically assisted births will have on representations of filiation. Effects of rupture between generations are necessary for the differentiation between generations, but in this case, these effects are particularly accentuated, and require some kind of resolution. (p. 8, translated for this edition)

We may no longer affirm, as we once did, that "you have only one mother" or that "pater semper incertus est, mater sed certissima". Reproductive techniques question these statements that possessed, until little more than thirty years ago, the quality of certainty throughout the generations preceding ours. However, genetic testing and the new architecture present in human fertility now make origins quite illusory.

To be born used to mean to be born from the body of a woman who was that child's mother. Among the effects of rupture and discontinuity in reproduction, nothing now guarantees biological bonds in reproduction. The last anchor point is not a woman's body, since a woman may now—paradoxically—be "looking at" her pregnancy and be present at her child's delivery if she rents a womb. Historically, women were always "in" their pregnancy.

However, beyond biology, the exercise of parenthood in the transmission of psychic life is based on maternal and paternal functions independent of the gender of the persons exercising them.

It is important to probe deeply into the place of bodies and desires in this field, in particular in cases of the donation of gametes—eggs and sperm—to differentiate what is one's own and what is the other's, in the categories of father and genitor and mother and genitor; in the same way, when a womb is rented, the way that maternity is divided into the maternity of a gestating woman and a "desiring" mother.

Contemporary maternities and paternities lead us to think that the desire to have a child is permeated by contexts of the day as well as cultural ideals and mandates transmitted throughout generations. These developments provoke questions in various directions in clinical work, some of these being the desire to have a child in men and women, the place of bodies and maternal and paternal functions, and the new origins with all the universe of meanings they acquire in each singular history.

A point to consider is whether we are simply dealing with a change of "clothing" in reference to the desire to have a child or whether new elements have entered with the new techniques and demands. For example, what place does a child occupy within the rules of kinship if his mother is his aunt, or if the child was gestated in her grandmother's womb or in the womb of a woman she will never meet. What are the projections on to this child? What place will the child be given by parental discourse and by discourse in the social field considering that both operate as matrices of identification references in the construction of a subject's identity?

Another question we need to consider is to what extent interventions to the body may be worked through and metabolised, since they mobilise fantasies originating in archaic representations. These are present in the infantile sexual theories, the primal scene, and the family romance of the neurotic (Freud, 1905d, 1909c).

The field of desire to have a child in men and women is, thus, embedded in epochal contexts presenting a new order in which sexual pleasure and procreation have been disconnected from the fertile period by radically dissociating sexual activity from reproduction. The way is open to determinants of desire, singular to each subject and tied to the traces of the subject's psychosexual development.

In the following sections, I develop some ideas, based on clinical observation, in reference to vicissitudes of the desire to have a child in women and in men, and offer some final reflections concerning the desire to have a child in relation to the new origins.

Vicissitudes of the desire to have a child

Desire to have a child is a central theme in parenthoods, as we have said. Each child has a history preceding that child that constitutes the prehistory of the child to be born; it is marked by what the child's real existence will represent afterwards for the parents' unconscious and projections (Alkolombre, 2008). It is also a product of the working through of an unconscious desire singular to each subject, inscribed in parental fantasies, imagos of infantile sexuality.

Conflicts and difficulties in accessing parenthood in men and women unfold in the course of clinical work in individual or couple treatments. The relation each patient establishes with reproductive technology is simply another element with which to work, since it may be at the service of accessing the maternal or paternal function or at the service of disavowal. This depends on the particular subjective position in each case.

Vicissitudes of the desire to have a child in women: the passion to have a child

Beginning in childhood, each woman creates complex networks concerning maternity, connected to the vicissitudes of her femininity, her history, and epochal context with its mandates and ideals.

At this time, maternity is not the only project given priority by many women. Many prefer to postpone maternity in order to advance in their occupational careers. In other cases, when they have not established a stable couple and the "biological clock" appears, they access maternity by means of a sperm donation.

Another vicissitude of maternity I discuss is linked to the notion of excess of drive. I was struck by the effort to achieve a pregnancy in women who were willing to do anything whatsoever to have a child. Many cases had a strongly sacrificial aspect, both because of the physical risk—having one assisted fertility treatment after the other—as well as because of economic risks they took, selling objects and properties in order to finance them. I could compare these cases to others in which they were starting to think about adoption or life without children. In the former cases, the child to come becomes an irreplaceable object, the receiver of maternal love. In clinical work, a profile began to take shape: the figure of the "child at any cost", a term coined by Delaisi de Parseval and Janaud (1983). This type is also associated with the idea of hypercathected maternity, in the manner of an obsessional idea, as described by Tubert (1991).

After a time, I began to think that it was a problem with narcissistic–passionate roots, as in couples with a passionate functioning: *you will belong to me or to nobody*. In this case, it is "I will have a child because I have to have one", in the words of Yerma, the protagonist of the eponymous play by García Lorca (1991, p. 77), in which she incarnates an indomitable determination to have a child.

I now present some fragments from an analysis that led me to begin to think about a narcissistic–passionate road in the field of the desire to have a child.

Marcela

Marcela is twenty-eight when she first comes to see me. She has been married to Ricardo for a year, and comments that she derives little satisfaction from their sex life. She is the middle sister of three girls, born a year after her elder sister, who was affectively closer to their mother, and before her first birthday her mother was pregnant again. She always kept her relation with her father distant. Throughout her session, she spoke of her desire to have a child and of her suffering; I tried to accompany her in understanding the roots of her complaint, the reasons for her strong fixation to the drive for pregnancy, as it related to her history and femininity.

Sometimes, we advanced in our understanding and she was able to decentre and to think of herself as someone fertile for life; however, after going forward, we went back over the same steps. The child was presented as an object of love with certain characteristics: unconditional, based on the foundational asymmetry in the mother–child link, and also a part of the mother's body, the seat of maternal narcissism. She repeated an almost identical discourse each month:

> This month I didn't get it . . . I'm not going to get it. Why does this have to happen to me . . .! Some women beg not to get it. Perhaps because of the obstacle the desire in me is greater. I don't know; I would have one after the other; it's the only thing that fills me, having babies. I would like to have many. (Alkolombre, 2008, p. 60, translated for this edition)

Her complaints also centred on her childhood history: having received less attention from her mother, there was little space for her as the middle daughter between two sisters; she had always felt left out.

Her associations and reflections are orientated initially towards the hypercathexis of the reproductive function, difficulties in her link with her mother, and increased castration anxiety, to explain the intensity of the affects involved, her difficulty in thinking, and the constant crises she suffered every month in view of the impossibility of becoming pregnant.

A year after she began analysis, she becomes pregnant with assisted fertility treatment, but her anxiety does not dissipate. She has now started to fear that her pregnancy is not developing well, that something untoward is happening.

She goes through the initial period of pregnancy with nausea and vomiting, revealing the ambivalence and anxiety with which she experiences this new condition. She gradually demands more and more of her mother: to help her with housework, to keep her company, even requiring her to wash her hair, since combing her own hair makes her feel nauseous. She begins to behave like a baby needing attention to her primary needs: she is now the baby to be cared for who cries out for her mother's presence. She tries to recreate part of her link with her mother, which was faulty in childhood, in the imaginary link with her child to come.

Throughout pregnancy, she was obliged to face and work through periods of great anguish and anxiety, which continued after her daughter's birth. Her desire to have a child in this case had two aspects: the narcissistic aspect, linked to her relation with her own body and her mother's body, and also the oedipal aspect in its inverted version, in which she struggles to capture her mother's attention by competing with her sisters. The father figure operates neither as a separator in the link with her mother, nor as reassurance of her feminine aspects; he is an absent father.

* * *

Clinical experience has enabled me to compare this case to others with characteristics similar to that of Marcela: perseverance in cruel and non-cruel testing, patients who underwent one treatment after another, many years invested, depressive states of greater or lesser intensity, and an excess of drive manifested in sacrificial and thanatic aspects associated with medical–technological treatments. However, two distinguishing characteristics in particular stand out: the fixedness or perseverance in this endeavour and its affective intensity. Other questions emerge: are these features explained only by the maternal ideal, female castration anxiety, and pre-oedipal conflicts (Freud, 1931b, 1933a, pp. 112–135).

This is the outset of a review that considers the withdrawal of libido and efforts to recreate a state of fusion with the originary object through maternity. We recall Freud's (1914c, p. 85) observation that when an individual falls ill, this person is less willing to love, and Freud adds that "in the last resort we must begin to love in order not to fall ill."

The passion to have a child is translated into living for a pregnancy; maternity is placed as part of the ideal—as something irreplaceable—that invites pleasure; as an absence, it generates intense suffering. In the words of Cournut (1999, p. 13), "passion is revealed in absence and in the subject's difficulty to work through the loss" (translated for this edition).

Consequently, I arrive at the hypothesis (Alkolombre, 2008) that

> in these women the desire to have a child is transformed into a passion to have a child: a unique object and recipient of this love. Passion is the form taken by the suffering of an ego that has submitted to the ideal of maternity. (p. 62, translated for this edition)

This passion emerges in the link with the absent child, fixed, incessant, boundless, and demanding. It is expectation signified by absence, establishing an inner dialogue with this lack, and constantly interrogating the body.

In the social imaginary, these maternities are associated to some extent with a desire that is typically considered naturally feminine. Although, in analytic listening, we find different theoretical lines and viewpoints, the desiring field of women is virtually totally saturated in maternity. Of the three destinies proposed by Freud (1931b) in the female Oedipus complex, the one leading to femininity is maternity.

I leave these issues open, together with the different perspectives concerning the psychosexual development of women, in order to probe more deeply into this topic, and to decentre the maternal as the only focal point of the destiny of femininity in women, with the child as her guarantor.

Paternity and the desire to have a child in men

Historically, we observe the hegemony of developments regarding the desire to have a child centred on women and maternity, supported biologically by anatomical difference; in psychoanalysis, the theoretical support that induces us, when we discuss the desire to have a child, to think of the resolution of the Oedipus complex in women and the symbolic equation, penis = child (Alkolombre, 2013). Psychoanalytic literature shows this interest centred on women and maternity.

When we investigate the subject of paternity, we find the ritual of *couvade*, in which the man takes the woman's place in the delivery. When the child is born, he takes the baby, gets into bed, and receives his neighbours' congratulations. This becomes the men's "delivery bed" and involves physical contact with the baby (This, 1982).

Always present in human preoccupations is male fertility. Male sterility is as old as humanity, and each culture seeks alternatives for its resolution. The first inseminations with donated semen go back three centuries (Frydman, 1986).

We may say that, in the context of contemporary parenthoods, both the broader panorama of paternity as well as the man's particular place in reproduction have become more complex and constitute a heterogeneous reality. We speak of paternities in the plural, traditional paternities originating in heterosexual couples and the new ones in male single parenthoods and single-sex parenthoods. A notable aspect is an increase in statistics of adoptions of children by single men (*La Nación*, 2010). Some paternities dispense with the female figure in their development, which is made possible by virtue of the application of two techniques of assisted fertility: the donation of ovules and womb rental.

These phenomena lead us to think psychoanalytically about elements made visible by these changes and to consider the greater desire to have a child in men. These roads lead us to a symbolic dimension of paternity and reveal the field of male desiring.

Concerning paternity, Delaisi de Parseval (1981) enquires what a father actually is, and notes that the answer is not so obvious; she proposes that we make visible the hidden part of becoming a father: is he the genitor, the educator, the mother's companion, or the wielder of the law?

There is an interesting paper by the historian Laqueur (1992), "The facts of paternity", in which he regrets that there is no history of paternity. He proposes that what is involved in being a man and being a father has been silenced, and also refers to the "emotional work" of paternity. To continue with this topic, we shall listen to some voices from clinical work.

Gustavo and Andrea

A couple, Gustavo and Andrea, consults me following the diagnosis of Gustavo's sterility. He had undergone surgery in infancy due to difficulties with undescended testicles and says that his parents had never talked to him concerning potential consequences to his fertility.

> Gustavo: Now I see black or white, I don't see greys. Why me! If I had known before, I don't know if I would have married ... I don't know; a child of one's own is something one wishes for, that one feels. I think about my parents ... one sees one's projection in one's children ... I have nobody to look at ... I feel that I have a very high wall and I can't jump over it.

Gustavo's words lead us to Freud's idea (1914c) concerning the double vicissitude of human beings, to be an end in oneself and also to be only a link in the generational chain. In this vignette, we observe the importance that blood ties, filiation, and the exercise of the paternal role have acquired: "to be the son of" and "to be the father of". They also reveal the suffering caused by the impossibility of transmitting his genetic material. Both members of the couple came from traditional families in which blood ties were cathected narcissistically.

Carlos and Adriana

Carlos and Adriana come to see me a few days after receiving a diagnosis of azoospermia. Following that announcement, Carlos began to suffer gastrointestinal symptoms: diarrhoea, gastritis, and reflux suggestive of the impossibility of "digesting" or metabolising this new reality.

Carlos: The doctor was too honest. This hit me like a bombshell . . . there are no spermatozoa . . . Who did I hurt! Who did I harm! [he says, looking at Adriana].

Adriana: He's depressive . . . but a year ago they tested him and it wasn't so bad! . . . I've never seen him like this . . . Yesterday he didn't go to work, he got sick last night, it started with a pain in his neck. He wept . . . (Alkolombre, 2008, p. 146)

Carlos symptomatically lost his identity documents twice; he also grew increasingly addicted to his work and more sombre. Neither of the two talked about it with friends or family; it was something they experienced with shame and grief.

The man's place in reproduction may represent a difficult crossroads. We are seeing problems that associate sterility with the castration fantasy and consequent anxieties that tie into the male Oedipus complex. Deprivation of the means of reproduction is experienced as successful castration, a punishment that reactivates castration anxiety and its derivatives. These experiences lead to analytic work with the desire to have a child in men.

This problem has been investigated very infrequently; the place of women in reproduction has always been the priority, the man's place remaining a true "black continent" (Alkolombre, 2001). This neglect is linked to the predominant place in culture of the ideals of masculinity, the man's place as genitor and companion of the mother, as provider and wielder of the law.

Although we find no references in Freud's works to men's desire to have a child, this search leads us into the territory of masculinity and male psychosexual development. In it, the father's function has a central role in the decline of the Oedipus complex, officiating as a third-party function in oedipal triangulation; a phallic function or paternal function, also called "the other of the mother", which operates in oedipal triangulation as a cut-off factor (Ceccarelli, 2007, p. 141).

The view associating only the feminine with the castrated has undergone revision and allows us to revisit the subject of masculinity from different clinical perspectives. In this direction, Nasio (1991) suggests that all those who must occupy the father's place need to recognise their "feminine part". He makes an interesting differentiation, since he distinguishes femininity from the neurotic man's idea of femininity, an idea that emerges from his castration anxiety. This anxiety refers to a synonym of passivity and submissiveness formulated in this way: "she suffers because she is castrated" (1991, p. 33, translated for this edition). However, he believes that when a man is able to accept his feminine part, breaking free from anxiety, and has been able to understand that there is a loss in any case, he may take on paternity, having gone through his fantasy of feminisation—the bedrock in men.

In child psychoanalysis, Aberastury (1984) discusses the notion of the wish to have a child in childhood, and considers that in boys the wish to have a child by their father in their belly is a normal wish in the first stages of the boy's development.

Taking up these ideas, we may rethink the idea linking aspects associated with the feminine in men is solely connected to their negative Oedipus complex, that is, their unconscious homosexual aspects, and open a way to think about the desire to have a child as an integral part of their masculinity.

These reflections led me to consider including in the paternal not only aspects of the masculine gender related to its more traditional profile, such as physical strength, sexual potency, and virility. We may include, without feminising it, the desire for paternity and to have a child in this largely unexplored field within psychoanalytic conceptualisations (Alkolombre, 2009).

The desire to have a child and the new origins

What is new and marks a difference is currently related to the origins, with reference to conditions of gestation that ushered in phenomena without precedent in history and require an effort of revision and investigation. There are now so many and such diverse ways to be conceived: sexual cells, fluids, and organs may be modified, permuted, and combined in different ways in order to access parenthood.

There is a new order in culture which radically separates sexual activity from reproduction and the ways to access parenthood. These roads present new articulations between blood ties, kinship, and filiation as a symbolic system.

Work on the desire to have a child considering the uncertainty of the origins unfolds in clinical practice, and I discuss some vignettes below.

Pedro and Karina come to see me when she is prescribed an egg donation. In the second interview, Pedro says to Karina, "I imagine you could feel strange with a pregnancy like that, as if you had an alien, you don't know where it comes from." The idea of the alien, a stranger or being from a different planet, brought up by Pedro, imposes itself forcefully on the session. It is a way to name, or draw with words, an outline of the presence of a donor in this gestation, an *unheimlich* aspect referring to the unknown within the familiar (Freud, 1919h).

Marta and Carlos, after undergoing several failed fertility treatments and various medical consultations, decided to resort to a sperm bank and ovule donation. In the middle of a session in the fifth month of pregnancy, a visibly anguished Carlos asks his wife, "What about the embryos? Where do they come from? There's a sort of gap . . . what are they like? What if it's Chinese?"

Formulated in this way, the question regarding the origins of the embryos, *Where do they come from? What are they like?*, we may conjecture their relation to another question that arises in childhood: "Where do children come from?" which comes with the awakening of the epistemophilic drive. Carlos's question—*what if it's Chinese?*—runs through the session and aims at the unspeakable of the unknown origins of the child they are expecting: a Chinese, a foreigner, a stranger. This idea is close to the idea of a "disquieting strangeness" (Aulagnier, 1992) in relation to births in which what is one's own is combined with something foreign in fertility. It leads us to the place of anonymous donors and the associated fantasies.

This clinical work contains many questions and the undetermined, especially when it is impossible to ascertain the biological source. Fantasies emerge: a Chinese man, an alien: words that allow us to outline the new origins and to represent the unknown.

We may say that these experiences are in tension between traditional parenthoods and the new ones. Novel accesses to parenthood expel us from the familiar ground of origins and sexuality, and, in analytic work with each case, the new origins open a universe with singular meanings.

To begin to conclude

In this chapter, I have set out on a path following the guiding thread of the desire to have a child in women, in men, and in relation to the new origins. In the intimacy of our consulting rooms we encounter individual patients or couples who consult when they are undergoing medical treatments, or those who, already in analysis, bring into play the desire to have a child with characteristics of the complemental series in each case and in each family and social context.

These complex problems present not only theoretical–clinical challenges, but also question the analyst's ideology in a field that brings together bodies and desires with different projects of parenthood.

As Leclaire (1992) points out, filiation is multi-determined and, therefore, cannot be reduced to a criterion of biological truth without including a "criterion of desire", referring to a symbolic order, and is tied into each subject's singular history.

These novelties test the analyst's permeability and openness to the new ways of being conceived, although analysts also know that every birth retains something enigmatic.

References

Aberastury, A. (1984). La paternidad. In: A. Aberastury & E. Salas (Eds.), *La Paternidad* (pp. 83–107). Buenos Aires: Kargieman.

Alkolombre, P. (2001). Esterilidad masculina, 'un continente negro' In: Segundas Jornadas de Infertilidad, Adopción y Fertilisación Asistida APdeBA (Eds.), *Fertilisación Asistida. Nuevos Avances, Nuevas Problemáticas* (pp. 11–15). Buenos Aires: APdeBA.

Alkolombre, P. (2008). *Deseo de Hijo. Pasión de Hijo. Esterilidad y Técnicas Reproductivas a la Luz del Psicoanálisis*. Buenos Aires: Letra Viva.

Alkolombre, P. (2009). Nuevos escenarios masculinos en fertilidad asistida: un vientre para él. In: M. U. Caplansky (Ed.), *El Padre. Clínica, Género, Posmodernidad* (pp. 153–160). Lima: Sociedad Peruana de Psicoanálisis.

Alkolombre, P. (2013). La paternidad y el deseo de hijo en el hombre: vicisitudes en los procesos de subjetivación. *Complejo de Edipo, 34:* 153–163.

Aulagnier, P. (1992). Qué deseo, de qué hijo. *Revista de Psicoanálisis con Niños y Adolescentes, 3:* 45–49.

Badiou, A. (1988). *L'Être et L'Événement*. Paris: Seuil.

Ceccarelli, P. R. (2007). Configuraciones edípicas contemporáneas: reflexiones sobre las nuevas formas de paternidad. In: E. Rotenberg & B. Agrest (Eds.), *Homoparentalidades. Nuevas Familias* (pp. 139–150). Buenos Aires: Lugar.

Cournut, J. (1999). L'Énergie de la passion. *De la Passion.* Paris: PUF.

Delaisi de Parseval, G. (1981). *La Part du Père.* Paris: Seuil.

Delaisi de Parseval, G., & Janaud, A. (1983). *L'Enfant à Tout Prix.* Paris: Seuil.

Freud, S. (1905d). *Three Essays on the Theory of Sexuality. S. E., 7:* 125–244. London: Hogarth.

Freud, S. (1909c). Family romances. *S. E., 9*: 235–241. London: Hogarth.

Freud, S. (1914c). On narcissism: an introduction. *S. E., 14*: 73–102. London: Hogarth.

Freud, S. (1919h). The "uncanny". *S. E., 17*: 217–256. London: Hogarth.

Freud, S. (1931b). Female sexuality. *S. E., 17*: 223–243. London: Hogarth.

Freud, S. (1933a). Feminity. In: *New Introductory Lectures on Psychoanalysis. S. E., 22*. London: Hogarth.

Frydman, R. (1986). *L'Irrésistible Désir de Naissance.* Paris: PUF.

García Lorca, F. (1991). *Yerma.* Buenos Aires: Losada.

Kaës, R. (2001). Transmisión entre generaciones: efectos de ruptura y efectos de solidaridad. *Transparencia, 3:* 8–9.

La Nación (2010). Cada vez más solteros adoptan chicos. 10 May, p. 10. Buenos Aires.

Laqueur, T. W. (1992). Los hechos de la paternidad. *Debate Feminista, Creación y Procreación, 6*: 119–141.

Leclaire, S. (1992). El criterio de verdad biológica: un apoyo rengo. *Revista de Psicoanálisis con Niños y Adolescentes, 3:* 56–60.

Nasio, J. D. (1991). La femineidad del padre. In: M. Alizade (Ed.), *Voces de Femineidad* (pp. 33–35). Buenos Aires: M. Alizade (self-published).

This, B. (1982). *Le Père: Acte de Naissance.* Paris: Seuil.

Tort, M. (1994). *El Deseo Frío. Procreación Artificial y Crisis de las Referencias Simbólicas.* Buenos Aires: Nueva Visión.

Tubert, S. (1991). *Mujeres Sin Sombra. Maternidad y Tecnología.* Madrid: Siglo XXI.

CHAPTER EIGHT

The role of the donor in assisted fertilisation treatments

Silvia Jadur, Viviana Wainstein, and Constanza Duhalde

Assisted reproduction techniques are legitimised in the collective imagination, as well as legalised in the field of public policy in many geographies. However, some bio-technological advances, such as egg and sperm donation and surrogate pregnancies, are still controversial. Since the topic is extremely broad, we narrow it down by highlighting some issues. We then address the donor's role in parenthood and its link with the subjective process undergone by those with reproductive disorders who need egg and sperm donation in order to become pregnant.

Gamete donation enables an individual or a couple who cannot conceive from their own eggs or sperm to become pregnant when receiving the gamete of another person, therefore resigning their own genetic transmission. When there is ovarian failure, early menopause, the after-effects of surgery, and in some situations where women have postponed pregnancy until fertility decreases, egg donation constitutes an option in order to conceive a biological child.

In any case, when a specialist in human reproduction diagnoses that the eggs have no reproductive capacity, both men and women are confronted with an arduous process of metabolisation. In our clinical practice, we often hear, "I never thought we could have these kinds of problems"; "It never occurred to us that I might not be able to get pregnant"; "I believed I was normal"; "We've always been careful, I never figured . . .". Likewise, when a man is informed of his azoospermia, both members of the couple suffer the impact and the effects of the lack of male reproductive cells. From the offset, the fantasy of a family with biological children is subsumed to uncertainty.

Mourning due to the loss of genetic illusion, the impact of the awareness of the lack of control and knowledge of the functioning of one's own body and the necessary subordination to the rules of biology, break up the "aspiration to mortality of the ideal ego".

The diagnosis of infertility, and, later, the possibility of gamete donation, put at stake and at risk the body's libidinal biography. This also reveals the individual's vulnerability and the fragility and narcissistic vicissitudes that emerge in such a situation. The difficulty of representing the "no-child" also appears at this stage in both members of the couple.

The possibility of elaboration offered by a psychotherapeutic setting provides a channel to representing in the long term, through the reproductive "failure-lack", the inclusion of a third person who opens another route to achieving biological parenthood.

As the psychic representation of time does not coincide with either biological or real time, it seems that the physician's word puts the individual in a position where the body adopts a dimension of vital presence by which individuals relocate themselves both in the world and towards themselves. The aging of eggs, for instance, is subsumed sometimes to the identity of the woman: the notion "I am old" also tears apart the illusion of eternal youth, and sets in motion the cycles and the finitude of vital processes.

Thus, the desire to be a parent has its transcription in the body. As far as the representation of a body subjected to the desire crumbles, the wounded narcissism dislocates the ego defences. The ego then takes shelter in the dysfunctional body, granting, at times, a new identity to the subjects. As a result, we can find individuals who introduce themselves as "infertile" as if this term were an identity definition. There is, as such, a libidinal reorganisation, a reinvestment of the body's self-image, an attention given to the awareness of the ailing self, together with a devalued feeling of the self.

Hence, the body puts affects to work, producing effects in the subjectivity and in the psychic economy. The *unheimlich* of the corporeal reality brings about uncertainty regarding whether a pregnancy will materialise, or a prospective child.

As well as patients gaining new knowledge of reproductive disorders and treatments and coming into contact with the scientific–medical discourse, pain opens up ignored subjective places, commonly filled with feelings that are unacceptable to them.

One of the intrasubjective tasks for these patients lies in accepting what is now unknown about that body which, as a trade-off, will have to accept the inclusion of an alien cell, the donated gamete, to conceive an infant. The disillusion of "natural" procreation is added to genetic resignation. This is a mandatory process of loss and an unavoidable mourning in order to build up the space required to offer a psychic site to the child.

It is indisputable today that women can make decisions about their bodies and desires, about their reproductive rights, from contraceptive care to the termination of a pregnancy, and especially about maternity. In this sense, egg donation, by offering the possibility of restitution of the failure in the body—the incapacity to produce a fertile egg—enables the woman to experience pregnancy, childbirth, and breastfeeding. The choice of this path towards motherhood permits her not to be resigned to the biological experience of motherhood.

We agree with Saal (1998) when she states that

> Each subject is talked about before its existence, he lives in projects and fantasies, fills up a space, absorbs libidinal energy, is a promise of being. That space is the mother's desire, and it is, also, a product of castration, which must not be reduced only to the singular desire of having a child, because motherhood is not the only function of women. What is proper of this desire, which makes motherhood a cultural act, not natural, as it has inappropriately been thought of, is the simple prerogative every woman has to say no to maternity. Under the possibility of a "no", a fundamental qualitative act is produced, which turns the act into a choice, not destiny. Giving life is not reduced to giving birth; giving life is becoming unattached. (p. 42, translated for this edition)

Langer, for her part, asserts: "In this past century women in our civilisation have acquired a sexual and social freedom completely unknown barely three generations back. However, cultural and economic circumstances impose serious restrictions on maternity" (1964, p. 13, translated for this edition).

Women possess a body ready for procreation, but the sociocultural situation, and even the mysteries of biology, influence the possibilities of choosing maternity and having it materialise. In some cases, the body is taken into account just as being responsible for reproduction. In such a case, the demand for a child assumes the shape of satisfaction of a need and, as a consequence, as Bydlowsky (1997) argues, the body is a generator of babies but it should be taken into account that the desire for a pregnancy does not imply by itself the desire for a child.

In this sense, Aulagnier (1975), sums up and organises the series of positions adopted by the proposition of the desire for a child in the psychic evolution of a woman through the oedipal trajectory. Furthermore, she puts forward the evolutionary hierarchy of the proto-identification and identification that place the being and the having in a dialectical relationship.

We see a difference, therefore, between desire for a child and the desire for maternity. Motherhood, as well as fatherhood, entails not only the desire, the medical treatment when necessary, pregnancy, and childbirth, but also sufficient availability in order to offer the child what it needs in order become a subject.

In order to lodge the embryos in the womb as a probability of the existence of a child, a process of intrapsychic work is required. This psychic work makes it possible to receive embryos made up of gametes (sperm–egg) that have been donated by another subject with a body and a history. We will borrow a philosophical term coined by Derrida (1967): "hospitality". This word derives from the Latin *hostis*, which means guest as well as enemy, the other. From this ambivalence, continuing with "host", in Spanish we use the term *huesped* to signify the guest received by the host. *Huesped*, the other, is the stranger, the not known, the unknown even by the nearest, the one who sometimes speaks another language though it might be the same, as long as there is always an alien dimension, alien and intimate in the other and the other in oneself.

In egg donation, the woman's body is on the stage. Therefore, the "hospitality of the woman's body" has a paradoxical effect. On the one hand, something inherently of her own is constituted, while, at the same time, lodging something alien. In fact, every pregnancy lodges another being, somebody unknown, an alien, a stranger ... Every embryo, as a potential future child, is a stranger that is lodged in the womb. It is crucial throughout this process that there is the possibility for the woman to invest in her own body and the womb, since this investing narcissistically will bring the suffering experience back to joy, pleasure, rather than tying it to psychic and physical pain.

We would like to point out that when we refer to an erogenous body, it is not from a biological standpoint, but in the real, symbolical, or imaginary registers. It is then that the ghosts of the oedipal drama act out the castration anxieties in face of the reality of the failed procreative function. The maternal identifications are, therefore, revisited and the non-fertility emerges as act/action of rivalry, competitiveness, and envy with the mother figure. The sense of "uselessness" present in the discourse of certain women might be linked to the incapacity to abide by the family reproductive design and the presence of a feeling of shame when the castration is revealed in face of the others' gaze.

In men, the discovery of a lack of spermatozoids in the initial test is rapidly intertwined with fantasies of loss of virility and male potency, self-esteem, and identity in relation to family and cultural mandates about progeny. When a sperm bank donation is considered so that a woman can become pregnant, the man is alienated from the biological circuit of procreation. The intra-subjective process does not only imply the genetic resignation but also implies being in charge of the paternity process. Paternal function is disengaged from biology. It does not mean either only to "give" the opportunity to the woman so that she does not miss her own biological and genetic perspectives. The issue, then, is how to make peace with an unmasked body and rebuild its deteriorated unconscious image. At the same time, it entails trying to build a family project prioritising the human bond rather than the union between an egg and a sperm.

The term "donor" (he/she), is already a global one (*donante*: Spanish; *donateur*: French), which is rather unfortunate from our point of view, since there is a symbolic economic compensation to him/her even if it is unprofitable, due to the work, time, and physical effort implied in this procedure. We suggest, therefore, the word "contributor" to refer to the man or woman who supplies the reproductive cells necessary to form the embryo.

In some countries, gamete donation is regulated by law; in others, it is done mainly through the recommendation of professional entities, and in others, it is banned.

Each specialised medical centre offers gamete donation programmes that are performed within a regulated and standardised clinical practice, detailing the required procedures for donors as well as recipients, which is not explained here. Instead, we underline the effects of the anonymity or otherwise of the donors and, especially, to reflect on the place assigned to them in the medical discourse and the patients' subjectivity.

As mentioned, every country has its own legislation regarding the anonymity or identification of the gametes' contributor. This has substantial implications for the patients' ability to receive gametes from an unknown person and for what will or will not be transmitted to a child about his or her procreative origin.

Let us agree on the fact that the donors will be neither the father nor the mother; they are just the genitors. They are those who supply the gametes, the ones who enable the recipients to be parents. They are the third parties who make up a history, a different conception—those who fulfil a crucial role in the new family. We might reflect here on several questions: would it be necessary for the child to know who the donor is? What would the child imagine about finding this person? Would it be a necessity or a curiosity? Would this need or curiosity belong to the parents or to the child?

Every infant possesses a natural epistemic concern about the origins of life and their own creation and birth. As long as the parents open up the space for knowledge, as long as sexuality is not conflicted for them, as long as donation has been processed, there should be a disposition to relate to the child the history of the family and the complexities of life. To build and transmit a narrative about life's origin constitutes a chance to resignify the vicissitudes of medical treatments, where the gamete contributors are part of the fabric that constitutes the child's subjectivity.

It is important to highlight that it is secrecy that we find problematic. That which is forbidden expression in words becomes a symptom even transgenerationally. It is the secret "towards the child" about how he or she was conceived, in this case with the gamete of another person, that should be avoided. The identity and/or identification of the donor does not play a necessary part in the knowledge of procreative origins. Would it be useful, necessary, and/or sufficient to identify the name or contact the donor in order to build the identity? Might that information be linked to a person's construction of identity, or drive a sense of curiosity?

Desire endows the psychic space and grants the child a symbolic place. His birth places the child as a singular person in his own cradle, and also as a subject inscribed in a lineage, in the community where he belongs. This means that for a child to exist, there must be at least one adult who has adopted a child symbolically as such, awarding him or her a place in the world. Here, again, we highlight the intention of receiving, lodging, a stranger. A presence of the unborn child manifests itself in parental dreams and family discourse. To focus on identifying donors means to displace parental desire and opportunity to accompany the child.

Follow-up research of families and their children has not reported any differences between families with children conceived by gamete donation. Problems will arise at each developmental stage, throughout any child's upbringing in any family, be it with the parents' own gametes, donated, or adopted.

At every stage of a child's development, parents are confronted with challenges. Those challenges are independent from the way children were conceived; problems arise during upbringing whether the gametes were donated or are a parent's own. The co-maternal families (female couples) or women who have chosen this path in order to be mothers and who do not have a partner, are usually the ones who talk to the children openly about donation. Even though we agree on the fact that communicating the truth to the child gives rise to safe and trustworthy bonds, families have the right either to inform their children on their procreative origin or not. A consideration of cultural idiosyncrasy, the original social sector, and the juridical–legal aspects on the issue generate respect and care towards the different actors: child, father, mother, contributor.

The journey that takes place towards the meeting of a child through assisted fertilisation treatment, especially gamete donation, need not be strictly traumatic. However, conflicts might arise when there are confusing or contradictory messages, or in situations where the child finds out that what s/he perceives is not supported by the grownups. One often hears about the child's right, the child's desire and its implications; here, we ask, what does a child need from a father, a mother, grown-ups, a community? We support Castoriadis's idea when he suggests that recovering the dimension of historicity entails a subjectivity that can think its present, past, and future.

It can be assumed that our Western civilisation is currently ruled by the formulae that mark the subjectivity of these times, characterised by speed, consumption, individual satisfaction, or the social and family requirements for success, even though human pain and distress still emerge daily. In the consultations of the people who have undertaken gamete donation as an option for becoming parents, the suffering related to the subject of time emerges as an imperative, involving the fear of the body's loss of control and the mourning of genetic continuity, all factors that erode libidinal energy.

The fact that, as analysts, we define our clinical work as a space for interrogation, enables the subjects to understand what otherwise might be called the "organic symptom", and explore different ways to reconnect with the desire for motherhood or fatherhood. This allows for neither placing the child as an object of satisfaction, nor as the means to restore broken narcissism.

It is pertinent in moving beyond the "necessary knowledge" to be capable of listening to the patient's demand, which, in many cases, is not a demand of analysis. We propose not to set ourselves up in competition with the medical discourse regarding the answers that patients seek. We insist on the personal enquiry, the case-by-case approach, situation by situation—even if various presentations might present common aspects.

The consultation associated with infertility and its medical treatment, particularly the donation of gametes, poses an imperative to think of new tools in clinical practice, not departing from the psychoanalytic postulates, but putting them to work from a different perspective, by means of perhaps flexible or less rigid frameworks.

It is important to bear in mind the numerous alternative medical proposals or psychological theories that are centred on behavioural guidelines, and the almost mechanical recommendations in order to avoid pain during treatment. Many "solutions" are offered that do not require an interrogative attitude from the subject but, rather, voluntary actions, where affects are quantified without their imbrication with the subject's history. These approaches do not create a subjective realm for a child to come, either from the parental desire or from the real "probability" that a pregnancy will occur.

The unexpected diagnosis/news of sterility does not necessarily imply a traumatic situation. The psychic structure can handle the deployment of the unconscious in different ways. The anguish, as a red light, announces an upsetting experience, opens an enquiry, allows the subject to essay the assembly of wishes and desires, taking into account both the impossibilities and the possibilities.

The brief passages of life experiences that we comment on are simple and frequent. They encourage in analysts and patients the use of creativity in order to deal with these demands that cannot be answered by medical–technical–biological speech.

Vignette: Maria and Pedro

They asked for an interview four years ago. They were referred by a physician, specialised in human reproduction, for a psychological consultation because he observed in them lasting anguish and fear in the face of the suggestion of egg donation.

Maria was forty years old at the time, Pedro thirty. They built a stable relationship through a slow process. They have been trying for a child for two years. At the end of the first year, as pregnancy did not occur, they sought a medical consultation. When confronted with the diagnosis, they decided to try assisted fertilisation, with a negative result. It took them two more years to collect the money required to make a second attempt, which was also unsuccessful. The post-treatment evaluation suggested the use of donated eggs in a future attempt to give them a chance to conceive because of low ovarian reproductive capacity due to Maria's age.

Maria needed some time to say it, to "whitewash" the relationship with a much younger man. They had met at work, and although the attraction was mutual, she felt uncomfortable with two important aspects of Pedro: his age, ten years younger, and his appearance, he is blond and fair-skinned.

Maria, who was born in the north of the country, is a beautiful woman with indigenous features: black hair and slanted eyes. Her husband is of German descent, very white skin and blue eyes. It had not been easy for her to leave her family life in the country. She has seven brothers; six of them are currently working with their parents as farmers, all with large families with many children. She is the only daughter, and the only one to come to the big city, Buenos Aires, far from home. She arrived when she was eighteen, to study at university, where she obtained her degree. "When I met Pedro", she says, "I was thirty-five. I thought that I was not going to start a family any more."

Maria: Sometimes I think that if God does not give me children it is because I do not deserve them. By coming to the city, I twisted my destiny.

Psychoanalyst: Twisting the destination?

Maria: Sure, it was assumed that I would marry a neighbour of my people, that I would help my parents ... And I am speaking here about this, it is difficult to me to deal with, something I cannot understand.

Psychoanalyst: You may think, perhaps, that you choose a different path, a different way.

Maria: Yes, that was Pedro's argument to convince me to start dating. He says when he met me he knew he wanted me to be his wife.

The analyst worked with the patient on the importance of decision making, the difference between choosing according to her wishes or following what she considered to be her destiny. Maria is a woman with strong religious traditions. She repeatedly refers to "what she deserves or does not deserve", the notion of punishment being very present in her speech.

Maria: How would I explain to my parents that my child has genes from another woman?

Psychoanalyst: It would be very difficult to accept that your child will have the genes of a donor, besides the ones of your husband.

Maria: I know that I'm going to love him—that carrying the baby in my belly will make me feel so close to him. But I fear that he will be white. Who guarantees that the donor woman has my skin colour?

Psychoanalyst: Even if the donor were your skin colour, are there guarantees? Even if they were your own eggs, would there be guarantees?

Maria: I know, but if my son is blond, I feel I betray my ancestors.

Psychoanalyst: Maria ... your husband is blond and has blue eyes, right?

While processing genetic resignation, Maria was dealing with aspects of family mandates, being a hazardous process to resign to the Ideal. Moreover, she felt that she kept transgressing: leaving her place of origin, the expectations on her as the only daughter, obtaining a university degree, choosing a different man and a different way to build a family . . .

At first, Maria thought that God was not sending children for some reason. Pedro had a strong desire to be a father, and, slowly, they evaluated together the options that science could provide. Eventually, they decided to accept treatment. Pedro agreed to do it from the beginning, Maria took longer. She was distressed about not knowing who gave the egg, the physical appearance of the egg donor, the colour of her skin.

Maria: I fear that when I meet the baby I will not recognise him as my son. I fear finding him very different from me.

Psychoanalyst: All children are different from us. What things do you think that genes transmit besides our appearance?

In this way the psychoanalyst and Maria worked on the differences between the genetic and the congenital, which is what parents transmit through words, affection, the difference between genetic identity and subjective identity. Also, who are the egg donors, if they were mothers, and so on. Step by step, Maria was able to prefigure the possible bond of a mother–infant relationship with her future son or daughter, to accept that conceiving is not the same as having children. Not to underestimate the important place of the egg donor, but to think that a child is part of the family of origin and integrate the child into their genealogical roots in a filiatory act. The couple could build a new frame, the family storyline.

Maria: I really fear having a white son. [She said in the first interview.] He is not going to have anything of my own, how will I take a blond son to my province? . . . I feel that I betray my ancestors.

These were statements which were resignified making a place for a child.

Maria and Pedro are now the parents of Lucas. Both families, over time, knew the history of procreation involving a donor. In periodic couple meetings, they related that the following words were part of their everyday dialogue, "A lady whom we do not know offered us an egg", "thanks to the help of the doctors you are with us".

Recently, they came back for some interviews because their child had started kindergarten. They are still putting together the history of the family, the story of expectation and desire for their child.

Vignette: Malena and Diego

Malena is thirty-two and Diego thirty-six. They have been living together for three years. When Diego was an adolescent, his father died of cancer. He then began to work with his eldest brother at the family company they had inherited. Meanwhile, their mother continued with her profession, supporting the home. His brother is married and has two children. They have a good working and fraternal relationship.

Malena's parents divorced when she was twelve years old. She and her two sisters lived together with their father. The elder sister is now married and has two children, the younger is single and soon became independent, moving away alone at the age of twenty-one. The parents' divorce came after an "eternally" violent relationship—the father had an aggressive and domineering style. Their mother met another man with whom she lived until he died. She works on her own and lives very humbly. Malena felt abandoned by her mother and does not have a good relationship with her.

It has been one year since they stopped using contraceptive methods and met a specialist in fertility. During the first week of the diagnostic studies, they were informed about Diego's definitive azoospermia of unknown origin. Diego was in psychotherapy from the moment of the diagnosis, and they also decided to engage in a psychological consultation as a couple.

In the second interview:

Diego: I am all right now. The penny dropped. Azoospermia, that's it. I have the option of the sperm bank or adoption. I want to be a father and have a family, that's something I've always wanted. My life was not easy, but not terrible either.

Malena: To adopt is not a possibility, I totally refuse. A time ago I did not think about having a child, but now, with Diego, yes. I want a baby now.

Diego: We can have a child, you can have it in your tummy, but not with my sperm. For me, the baby will be our child and I will be the father. I want to see you with a tummy. I look ahead. I always had to fight and I got what I proposed to get. There is a way to solve the problem; it's not what I wanted, but I've already cried, and thought about what is most important.

Malena: I feel worse than him. He is optimistic. I am very afraid of not being able to connect with the boy. I wanted our child!

Diego: But the baby will be ours.

Malena: I do not know who the sperm donor is ... who will the baby look like ... He won't look like you. When I look at the baby, whom will I be seeing?

We decided to have interviews with Malena twice a week. The topics addressed were the relationship with her mother, the importance of approaching her and giving up the idea of an ideal mother from an infantile position. She was able to talk about the history of her parents' divorce, her fantasies about motherhood, and desires and fears.

Malena: I cannot imagine me with a belly. They will place the sperm of someone in my body whom I do not know and I will not know. I will not be able to recognise Diego's gaze in the eyes of the baby. This was not expected. The worst thing is that Diego is fine with it. I cannot believe it. And it's me who feels awful ... It was a great help to him to talk with his mother; she said, "What is the problem?! The baby will be my grandson or my granddaughter. What is the problem? Children should always be welcome in this world."

After this talk with the mother, Diego felt reassured and changed his mood.

Gradually, both of them were able to process the acceptance of sperm donor insemination treatment. In his analytic space, Diego could resignify his own father's loss in order to feel enabled in his non-genetic paternity. After further couple consultations, they decided to get married. This project is a first step on their path to building a family, from where they can interweave the desire for a child, maternity–paternity, with the participation of a third donor party.

In our clinical task, we continue learning, generating questions, and building bridges between psychoanalysis and the advances in human reproductive sciences.

References

Aulagnier, P. (1975). *La violence de la interpretation. Du pictogramm e a l'ennoncé.* Paris: Presses Universitaires de France.

Bydlowsky, M. (1997). *La dette de vie.* Paris: PUF.

Derrida, J. (1997). *Hospitalidad* (Hospitality). Buenos Aires: Ediciones de la Flor.

Langer, M. (1964). *Maternidad y sexo* (Motherhood and Sex). Buenos Aires: Paidos.

Saal, F. (1998). *Palabras de analista* (Analyst's Words). México City: Siglo XXI.

CHAPTER NINE

Parenthood for same-sex couples and gender definition in children

Eva Rotenberg and Beatriz Agrest

> "In scientific affairs there should be no place for recoiling from novelty. Science, in her perpetual incompleteness and insufficiency, is driven to hope for her salvation in new discoveries and new ways of regarding things . . . [Scepticism] may be sharply directed against what is new while it spares what is familiar and accepted, and it may be content to reject things before it has examined them"
>
> (Freud, 1925e), p. 213)

Introduction

In the twenty-first century, the organisation of the family has changed significantly from what used to be considered a unique format: father, mother, and children. Nowadays, we come across different types of families, such as adoptive, extended, and foster families, single parents, unmarried couples, heterosexual couples, same-sex parents. In addition, there are yet other couples who originally belong to the same sex but, from the perspective of the imaginary, one of their members identifies with the opposite sex and carries out transformations, as in those cases where "the woman" is a transvestite or a transsexual, among other forms of family construction.

Parenthood for same-sex couples

The position of the analyst today, faced with the social, cultural, and scientific metamorphoses of the present century, leads him to examine these transformations and their effects. Among them, the issue of same-sex parenting is controversial both socially and among psychoanalysts. It invites agreements and disagreements and, what is more, there is no consensus about it in all cultures.

In order to approach the different aspects of same-sex parenting from a psychoanalytic perspective, we embarked on a theoretical and clinical exploration in 2000 with a study group called "Adoption, Same-sex Parenthood, and Sexual Diversity", at the Argentine Psychoanalytic Association, which we chaired.

These studies led, in turn, to encounters and theoretical–clinical exchanges with colleagues from the IPA, who held different opinions about this subject. It was at the IPA Congress in Rio de Janeiro (2005) where we presented the first workshop on the subject. From then on, the presentations continued, awakening both keen interest and controversy within the psychoanalytic community.

In 2007, we gathered these important exchanges carried out with colleagues from different countries and positions in a book titled *Homoparentalidades. Nuevas Familias* (Same-Sex Parenthood), followed by a second edition in 2010.

This book was consulted by the Commission of the Legislative Body, before the promulgation of the same-sex marriage law in Argentina.

Since the 1970s, several sociological and psychological research projects were carried out in the USA and the UK. They used different variables, such as behaviour, sexual orientation, and social inclusion, which were studied in the children of lesbian couples, who, then, were the ones who predominated within same-sex parenting. Among these projects there is one in particular that we would like to mention about the sexual orientation of adolescents, which was based on the comparative study between the children of lesbian couples and those of heterosexual couples. Results showed that the proportion of heterosexual object choice was higher in both groups and, equally, lower was the proportion of homosexual object choice in both groups (Golombok & Tasker, 1996).

With the ideas presented by different authors and disciplines, such as anthropology and sociology, other possibilities of parental configurations have become known, where more than two people play a part: co-parenting, pluri-parenting, which are configured according to the singular decision and the wish for a parental project on the part of their members, thus configuring *homoparentalité*, as they have been termed in France (Cadoret, 2003).

One of the forms of parenting, "same-sex parenting", is a reality that has been silenced for years, as the numerous consultations sought by divorced parents who have then come out and established homosexual or lesbian relationships amply show.

What is nowadays new is that the legalisation of the homosexual civil unions has granted legal status to what was previously considered as "marginal", therefore granting these unions the same rights that heterosexual couples enjoy.

At present, it should be acknowledged that there is a sexual diversity that cannot be reduced to the "male–female" binary classification, or to homosexuality and lesbianism. There is, in fact, sexual diversity: transvestite, transsexual, transgender individuals, and the so-called "migrant sexualities". However, in this chapter, we confine ourselves to studying same-sex parenting.

Homosexuality and the changes in its conceptualisation in psychoanalysis

Homosexuality can hardly be considered univocal; therefore, we prefer to make reference to homosexualities, in the plural, which, along with heterosexualities, are included in a broad psychopathological range, of a varied nature, that includes people of different sexual orientations. In this way, heterosexuality and homosexuality are regarded as different object choices and, thus, homosexuality is separated from perversion, which can manifest itself in different individuals beyond their sexual object choice.

Indeed, homosexuality does not involve paedophilia as certain preconceptions claim: there is a social prejudice that children are sexually abused by homosexuals. Rather, paedophilia is a sexual perversion frequently found among different sexual orientations (American Psychiatric Association, 2013).

Goldberg (2001) asks what depathologising homosexuality means. He suggests that, according to Freud, surmounting the Oedipus complex is complicated, and that this complexity should be taken into account in each and every individual, beyond his or her sexual orientation.

From the perspective of Silvia Bleichmar (2007),

> The position taken on same-sex parenting is closely connected to that on homosexuality. If the latter is considered a perversion, there is no doubt that same-sex parenting will not be regarded with a friendly eye. There is no unified position on this issue in psychoanalysis because within it different theories coexist, which, in turn, grant different value to the anatomical sexual differences and manifest different opinions about the oedipal. (p. 91, translated for this edition)

Considerations about perversion

At present, a univocal conception of the notion of perversion can hardly be considered. Following Kernberg's ideas (2001), homosexuality can no longer be included within the group of perversions because perversions, from a clinical perspective, are characterised by a restriction of the individual's sexual inclination to a partial, perverse sexual drive that dominates his whole sexual behaviour.

There is, nowadays, a current within philosophy and psychoanalysis that characterises perversion as the de-subjectivation of the other to inconceivable limits, as the object might not even be considered as a fellow human being. The other and his or her body are made use of without their consent. Thus, there is an exercise of power and cruelty over the other, who ends up being dehumanised.

A further idea put forward by Bleichmar (2007) is quite interesting:

> The Oedipus complex, either positive or negative, marks the moment when partial sexuality becomes reunited in the love towards the other and, in this sense, constitutes a moment of binding and sublimation. Therefore, I consider that homosexual or heterosexual love is part of the road towards the possibility of establishing a relationship with a

> fellow human and linking eroticism and tenderness. I am more concerned with the deadly aspects of the dehumanisation of the other that manifest themselves through pseudo-genital forms—to put it in Melanie Klein's words—as the body is taken as an object deprived of subjectivity. It is there where true perversion lies. (p. 93, translated for this edition)

We believe it is appropriate to consider that nowadays sexuality, either in its homosexual/lesbian or heterosexual forms, could be considered as a perversion when it presents the characteristics of pregenital fixation, polymorphous migration, and the de-subjectivation of the other.

How the Oedipus complex should be considered within same-sex couples

The primary and secondary identifications, and the sexual orientation of the child, depend on the relationship between the parents, whichever their sexual orientation, on their unconscious desires, traumas, defence mechanisms, and transgenerational identifications, which all manifest themselves in the pre-oedipal and oedipal stages.

As to the Oedipus complex, which was conceptualised by Freud based on the unique model of the heterosexual nuclear family, in the triangular structure of which the father takes the central role as the Law, it is essential that it is revisited.

According to Deleuze and Guattari (1972), the Oedipus complex imposes on its three members a fixed, definitive position. Nadeaud (2002) concurs with this notion that the Freudian complex is both universal and immobile and points out, too, "the existence of several relationships within the multiplicity of families, that is, the different Oedipus complexes" (Deleuze and Guattari, quoted in Nadeaud, 2002, p. 40, translated for this edition).

In view of the socio-cultural transformations, we consider that the Oedipus complex should be considered not only in its double identificatory–identifying relationship with both parents, but should also include the sibling complex. Indeed, given the multiplicity of parental configurations in Western civilisation, it should be constantly reviewed and questioned within contemporary psychoanalysis, beyond the traditional family core.

We should consider how the Oedipus complex comes to be surmounted, and the way in which the connection between infantile sexuality and the symbolic castration is produced within the context of an affective parental bond.

The wish for a child and access to parenthood nowadays

The wish for a child condenses different conscious and unconscious representations that stem from the pre-odipal and oedipal infantile relationships within the context of the complemental series.

According to Aulagnier (1975), this concept undergoes a series of transformations: to be the object of the mother's desire, to want to have a child by the mother, to accept the difference between the sexes, to want to have a child by the father, to give a child to the father, and, from the time when one becomes a mother, to wish that one's own child should become a father or mother.

Until not so long ago, it was assumed homosexuality involved relinquishing, and grieving, both consciously and unconsciously, the project of having children. This has changed, not only because scientific progress has made possible the separation, unthinkable before, between procreation and intercourse, but also because there is higher tolerance of lesbian and homosexual parenting.

However, the wish for a child could appear once the imaginary impossibility has been worked through both intra-subjectively and intersubjectively, and this includes giving up the wish to have a child *between* the members of the couple. We could say that biology, today, is not destiny.

Gay and lesbian couples have different approaches to parenthood, although the wish for a child could be equally important for both members of the couple. This is why we should revise the symbolic equation described by Freud in women: penis–faeces–babies.

Men also wish to have children and, in both sexes, the wish for a child involves a wish for the transcendent, and the passage of generations. However, not everyone wishes for a child.

Same-sex couples present we analysts with new theoretical and clinical uncertainties about parenthood and its vicissitudes, as well as the subjective development of the children. For all this, we consider that the interchange and follow-up among colleagues is essential.

In the case of a lesbian couple, both women had become pregnant via artificial insemination. They consulted because each felt that the baby each had been pregnant with was "more their own child", than the other child. This was interfering with their relationship as a couple and as a family. This vignette illustrates the singular conflicts that appear in some of these couples, as explored by Vaughan (2007).

Other authors have made reference to the "family function" and its adequate performance, which could allow for the construction of an inner family, satisfactory enough for the symbolic development of the child (Alizade, 2007), thus considering the potential of all human beings to cathect the other, to look after a child, and to replace an inadequate family.

Homosexuals can nowadays become parents by means of the possibilities offered by the ever-developing assisted fertilisation techniques: surrogacy arrangements, sperm donors who might or might not later play a role in parenting, among others. With regard to adoption, and depending on the legislation in force in each country, same-sex couples usually face more obstacles than heterosexual couples or single people.

Lesbian women usually decide which member of the couple will become pregnant, whether the donor will be anonymous or not, or whether the pregnancy will be achieved by means of intercourse. They might also have children from previous marriages.

These forms of access to parenthood have not yet become legalised in all countries, and many judges still consider that the biological bonds are of greater importance than the affective ones.

We believe that this requires an interdisciplinary work that takes ethics into account, so that future parenting is a true encounter between parents and their children.

The different ways children identify with gender, which might or might not coincide with their biological sex

On the definition of gender identity in children

In our clinical practice, we noticed that, until not so long ago, homosexuals and lesbians were the children of heterosexual couples, which led us to explore the way in which gender identity could be assumed beyond the sexual definition of the parents. Hence, we could ask ourselves, do the children of same-sex couples have limited options in their identification models?

The different vicissitudes of the processes of identification in children might lead them to assume a certain gender identity that may or may not coincide with their biological sex.

We consider that identifications with the parent of the same sex are neither lineal nor direct; rather, they have to do with the surmounting of the broadened Oedipus complex, with the unconscious, with infantile psycho-sexuality, and with the transmission across generations (Rotenberg, 2014). We should also take into consideration the identification with the fantasies of the parents, as well as the experiential intertwining that is generated within "the reciprocal interdependence between parents and their children" (García Badaracco, 1985).

In addition, starting from the dissolution of the Oedipus complex, we should take into account all four aspirations included in it, revising the concepts of perversion and parental functions.

Fast's (1984) theory of gender differentiation argues that children are initially bisexual, thus reinterpreting the idea of bisexuality to mean not a constitutional biological anlage, but a position of identifying with both parents. In the pre-odipal phase, children are "over-inclusive": they believe they can have or be everything. During childhood, children do not recognise the exclusivity of the anatomical difference; they want what the other sex has, not instead of, but in addition to, what they have (Benjamin, 1995).

Before the anatomical sexual differences are established, there are other categories of difference that constitute subjectivity, such as the difference between generations, the acknowledgement of the child as an other, and, following Benjamin, the difference in both gender equality and gender difference. The child, whether boy or girl, acknowledges the mother as an other with her own desires. In fact, Benjamin, on freeing herself from the phallic reference in order to explain the process of rupture of the mother–child symbiosis, contributes with a change of perspective.

In the Freudian thought, however, there is no primary femininity, but, rather, just one genital: the phallus. Therefore, it would seem that there is no direct access to the notion of difference (Glocer Fiorini, 2001).

Interesting contributions are those made by Bleichmar (2007), who, within the context of identifications, analyses if the father acknowledges and responds to the masculinity or the femininity of the boy and the girl, respectively. She claims that the masculine and the feminine identities are mainly determined by the identification with the conscious and the unconscious attitudes of the adults towards their children. According to the nature of these attitudes and affects, there could be, or not, disturbances in the construction of what she has termed the child's "sex–gender system".

We think, therefore, that there might be another category of "difference", which is the acknowledgement of the parents, who offer back a passive identifying gaze that is often previous to any object relationship.

With regard to gender identity in children (whether it is consolidated or not), an issue that causes us much concern is the treatment offered to those boys and girls who claim they feel they belong to the other gender. What does the analyst listen to in cases such as these? Will the child's future be the same if he is in treatment with an analyst with little training in these issues or with another, fully trained and free from prejudice (or not)? Hence, we think it is essential to analyse the relationship between the concepts of "parental function, anxiety, and gender identity", the "professional function", and the ethical position of the analyst.

We have seen boys in treatment because their parents were concerned by the fact that they felt they were girls, and also girls who claimed they were lesbians. Although these treatments developed in their own unique ways, what was approached in all of them was the children's own identifications, those of the parents, the desires of two generations, the fantasies, and the role played by the parents' mechanism of disavowal throughout their infantile and transgenerational history.

Freud introduces the uncanny (1919h), and his speculation leads him to the intrapsychic, to "the demonic character", the neurotics' feeling of guilt.

Marucco (1999) reviews the Freudian ideas about trauma and asks himself who is threatening the destruction of the ego and whether it could be the omnipotence of death, or rather the action of the "desire" (traumatic situation) of "another" at the very beginning of the structuring of the ego? This idea leads to the notion of a non-repressed, split off unconscious system, "the double", which comes into being through the desires and the yearnings of "the others", the effect of which is the mechanism of disavowal.

At this point, we would like to emphasise that, although the effects of the complemental series on the psychic structuring continue to hold full validity, we think that the actual effects on the child of the desire of the other, with its drives and its traumas, has been overlooked. In certain cases, it goes way beyond the narcissistic cathexes of the parents and, depending on the degree of parental disavowal, might even be acted out on the child and his body.

For instance, we once attended a congress where an analyst presented a clinical case. A six-year-old boy, who said he felt he was a girl, was seen by an interdisciplinary team and the doctors prescribed feminine hormones, a change of identity card, of name, and of school. Thus, we are faced with the abject. The abject is literally to operate on the body of a child whose sexual identity might not yet be assumed. Can the child's ego metabolise these changes? Or is it, rather, an act of intrusion on a child who lacks a sufficiently developed psychic apparatus that can allow him to work through the actions affecting him?

Whose desires are at stake here? Is it the desire of the parents, or of the analyst? Could it be the desire of the doctors? Or is the desire of the child already structured?

With regard to the abject, Kristeva (1988) establishes a distinction between the uncanny and the abject. Freud (1919h) uses the term *Heimlich*, which, in German, has two different meanings, one of which coincides with *unheimlich*. On the one hand, *Heimlich* refers to the familiar, and, on the other, to the occult. The uncanny, as in "The Sandman", leads us back to the anxiety provoked by the infantile castration complex (that involves an intrapsychic process, an identification complex, and object choice).

The distinction between the abject and the uncanny pointed out by Kristeva is that the abject is more violent; there is nothing familiar about it, as it is built on the failure to acknowledge the child's true self and on the parents' desire for power.

In some of these cases, others take control of the child's decision; they take control of the desire of a child whose ego runs the risk of transforming into a parental fetish because it has suffered the effects of the parental splitting and disavowal. Thus, we could say that the child is spoken by others, as it were, not only in the intrapsychic dimension, but also in the intersubjective one.

If the actual action of identity change is carried out, he then becomes trapped, alienated, as the child is forced to take the position of the ideal ego, the fetish. We should stress that this is the case even if the child is really determined to change his identity on reaching adulthood.

In this way, the subjectivity of the child is disturbed and his true self cannot develop. The decision to administer hormones becomes concealed by the so called "desire of the child".

Thus, what would appear to be the acknowledgement of what the child has expressed (offer him hormones) is, in fact, an act of perversion. This action upon the body of an underage child constitutes a transgression that involves the mechanism of disavowal, where one or more adults take possession of the child's body. This takes place before the child has reached an age when his feelings and experiences can gain meaning for him, before his ego becomes capable of working through all the possible changes.

The desire can only be sustained by an ego that has been able to master his own feelings, to integrate his own psyche–soma, his emotions. In contrast, it can never be sustained if another takes possession of his own desires. The origins of the abject lie precisely there and we, in our capacity as analysts, should have our say in this regard.

Through the abject, an important failure in the parental function is expressed: perversion, where the one who should perform parental functions fails to accept the symbolic castration. It is a perverse or a psychotic act that we are dealing with here, an action that has effects on the constitution of the child's subjectivity. In addition, there is a failure in the categorisation of difference on the part of the adult.

Parental function

It is important to remark that parental functions do not necessarily have a direct interrelationship with the biological sex of the members of the couple.

In fact, we consider that both the mother and the father should be able to acknowledge His Majesty the baby, the child of narcissism, as an other, and they themselves should operate as a third instance, as they have experienced incompleteness.

In same-sex couples, or different-sex couples, one of the members "might exercise thirdness, while the other carries out its nurturing function and both functions can be shared and/or interchanged" (Rotenberg, 2014, p. 39).

Thus, reconsidering parental functions allows us to question the myth claiming that heterosexuality is the guarantor of children identified with their own biological sex, or of healthy children.

This position involves a psychic demand because there is need for a change in the social imaginary that, from the very origins of culture, has remained fixated to biology. Even from the Biblical myth of Adam and Eve, a man and a woman are needed to have children. However, what is actually needed in order to conceive children are eggs and spermatozoon. To conceive does not mean to be a parent who exercises his/her functions, and parents need not be of a different sex.

Winnicott (1960) developed the concepts of true and false self in children. In our clinical practice, we confirmed that many of the children who had constructed a false self when they were children became, in turn, "as if" parents when they reached adulthood, that is, they felt unable to support their children and to develop a safe attachment.

We use the term "true self parental function" (Rotenberg, 2014) to refer to the function that allows the child to experience "a continuity of being" (Winnicott, 1960).

If the baby can count on a significant other who validates his perceptions, feelings, and needs, he is allowed not only to experience illusion, but also the integration of psyche–soma and ego. The "true self parental function" would be the possibility on the part of the adults of carrying out the functions of attachment, emotional support, and thirdness within an intrapsychic and intersubjective relationship.

The mother as mirror is a metaphor that shows that the ego has an imaginary aspect, that it constitutes a narcissistic object involving drives and their vicissitudes, as well as the other with his own drives.

This imaginary gaze might affect the early determination of gender. The ego is connected to the experience and to the presence of the other; the self emerges when the child realises who he is through the gaze of the other (Winnicott, 1960).

If the other reflects in a distorted way, what does the child see in that gaze? How could his identity be constructed? This leads us to consider the disturbances in certain parental functions and their effects.

A good enough upbringing involves helping to build the emotional set-up in such a way that the child is able to internalise emotional encounters experienced through an acknowledgement of his being. It is "a way of conceiving the internal set-up, taking the encounter with the others as a starting point", "normogenic identifications structure the individual's ego resources, while pathogenic identifications constitute relationships that force the self to transform in order to satisfy the desire of the other (García Badaracco, 1985, pp. 504, 510, translated for this edition).

Filiation

Derrida and Roudinesco (2001) suggest that the advances in research in fertilisation will confront us in the future with plural origins. This leads us to approach the concept of filiation, a concept of legal and anthropologic roots that, along with the changes in the parental configurations, has broadened its conceptualisation. At the moment, there are different categories of the concept of origin that could support the notion of filiation, which also requires being reviewed and updated.

The basis of filiation has been viewed as stemming from a legitimised union, the imposition of a name such as the different societies define it, to offer legitimacy to a child, the filiation to a group, the first symbolic net, as proposed by Françoise Heritier (1992).

In same-sex couples, blood relationships, one of the axes defining filiation within the traditional family, are replaced by the affects that led them to desire, conceive, or adopt their children. Thus, the concept of filiation linked to blood relationships changes.

The relationships between the parents and their children are based on the intertwining between the parents' subjectivity and their desire, which symbolically, and previous to the advent of the child, will mark the origins of this child. We agree with Bleichmar, who also emphasises the symbolic origin, which converges in the welcome achievement of the affective and psychic filiation.

With regard to the children and their knowledge of their origins, we face diversity once again. If we are dealing with legal adoptions, the account of the child's origins becomes facilitated. In addition, adolescents have a right to know about their origins. On the other hand, there are differing voices regarding what to disclose when we deal with children born with the help of assisted reproduction techniques. Nowadays, due to the diversity of treatments and their increasing complexity, referring to the children's origins appears to have become more difficult both for couples and single parents. For this reason, an interdisciplinary analysis will probably be necessary for each unique case.

In agreement with many of the authors referred to in this chapter, we believe that spontaneity and transparency, honesty, and an ethical attitude are all essential when it comes to telling children about their origins (Agrest, 2007, 2014).

The child has a right to know about his origins, to obtain an identity, to acknowledge, and give new meaning *après coup*, to his own history. From another perspective (Agrest, 2007) Golombek also agrees with the account given to a child about his origins. In his findings, we read that both gay fathers and lesbian mothers are in favour of the transparency in the communication of their children's multiple origins.

Final words

We have approached complex issues about same-sex parenting, gender definition in children, and filiation, which is based not only on biology, but also on the scientific progress that affects the individual and his origins.

An essential issue to be considered is the ethics of the analyst and science. All these considerations lead us to constantly review contemporary psychoanalysis, such as Freud himself did until the end of his life.

References

Agrest, B. (2007). Homoparentalidades, adopción y filiación. In: E. Rotenberg & B. Agrest (Eds.), *Homoparentalidades. Nuevas Familias* (pp. 121–126). Buenos Aires: Lugar.

Agrest, B. (2014). Padres del mismo sexo y parentalidad. In: E. Rotenberg (Ed.), *Parentalidades* (pp. 275–289). Buenos Aires: Lugar.

Alizade, M. (2007). Homoparentalidades. In: E. Rotenberg & B. Agrest (Eds.), *Homoparentalidades, Nuevas Familias* (pp. 77–83). Buenos Aires: Lugar.

American Psychiatric Association (2013). *The Diagnostic and Statistical Manual of Mental Disorders (Volume 5) (DSM-5)*. Arlington, VA: American Psychiatric Association.

Aulagnier, P. (1975). *La violence de la interpretation. Du pictogramme a l'ennoncé.* Paris: Presses Universitaires de France.
Benjamin, J. (1995). Sameness and difference: toward an over inclusive model of gender development. In: *Like Subjects, Love Objects* (pp. 49–79). London: Yale University Press.
Bleichmar, S. (2007). Las nuevas cuestiones ponen en crisis viejas teorías, E. Rotenberg interviews S. Bleichmar. In: E. Rotenberg & B. Agrest (Eds.), *Homoparentalidades. Nuevas familias* (pp. 91–98). Buenos Aires: Lugar.
Cadoret, A. (2003). *Des Parents comme les autres. Homosexualité et parenté.* Paris: Odile Jacob.
Deleuze, G., & Guattari, F. (1972). *El Antiedipo.* Barcelona: Barral.
Derrida. J., & Roudinesco, E. (2001). *De quoi demain* (pp. 43–55). Paris: Librerie Artheme Fayard et Editions Galilee.
Fast, I. (1984). *Gender Identity: A Differentiation Model.* Hillsdale, NJ: Lawrence Erlbaum.
Freud, S. (1919h). The "uncanny". *S. E., 17*: 217–252. London: Hogarth.
Freud, S. (1925e). The resistances to psychoanalysis, *S. E., 19*: 213–222. London: Hogarth.
Garcia Badaracco, J. (1985). La identificación y sus vicisitudes en la psicosis, y la importancia del concepto de objeto enloquecedor. *Revista de Psicoanálisis, 42*(3): 504–510.
Glocer Fiorini, L. (2001). *Lo femenino y el pensamiento complejo.* Buenos Aires: Lugar.
Goldberg, A. (2001). Depathologizing homosexuality. *Journal of the American Psychoanalytic Association, 49*: 1103–1480.
Golombok, S., & Tasker, L. (1996). Do parents influence the sexual orientation of their children? Findings from a longitudinal study of lesbian families. *Developmental Psychology, 32*: 3–11.
Heritier, F. (1992) Del engendramiento a la filiacion. In: *Revista de Niños y Adolescentes no 3* (pp 22–31). Buenos Aires, Argentina.
Kernberg, O. (2001). Aspectos controversiales en la teoría psicoanalítica de la homosexualidad y Bisexualidad, in Trópicos, 1, XI, Caracas, English version available: "Unresolved issues in the psychoanalytic theory of homosexuality and bisexuality".
Kristeva, J. (1988). *Poderes de la Perversión.* Madrid: Siglo XXI.
Marucco, N. (1999). *Cura analítica y Transferencia.* Buenos Aires: Ed. Amorrortu.
Nadeaud, S. (2002). *Homoparentalité, un nouvelle chance pour la Famille?* Paris: Fayard.

Rotenberg, E. (2014). La función parental verdadero self base de la integración del yo de los hijos. In: E. Rotenberg (Ed.), *Parentalidades, interdependencias transformadoras entre padres e hijos* (pp. 37–69). Buenos Aires: Lugar.

Vaughan, S. (2007). Scrambled eggs. *Journal of Infant, Child and Adolescent Psychotherapy, 6*: 141–155. Reprinted as: Huevos revueltos. In: E. Rotenberg & B. Agrest (Eds.), *Homo parentalidades. Nuevas Familias* (pp. 149–163). Buenos Aires: Lugar, 2010.

Winnicott, D. W. (1960). The theory of the parent–infant relationship. In: *The Maturational Processes and the Facilitating Environment* (pp. 33–55). New York: International Press.

CHAPTER TEN

Are we pregnant? Fantasies displayed in the embryo transfer process

María Alejandra Rey

Introduction

Are we pregnant? That was the question Sonia asked herself when they carried out the first embryo transfer.

Married to Miguel, ten years ago they decided to try to have their first child and it was then that they found out that she did not ovulate. Their doctor recommended that they follow a course of programmed intercourse (this technique consists of monitoring the development of ovulation to determine the optimum moment for the couple to have sexual relations and thus increase the probability of achieving pregnancy) and, at their first attempt, she became pregnant and Carolina—presently five years old—was born. Sometime later they decided to try and have a second child. They tried four times with programmed intercourse, were not able to conceive, and so passed on to the second stage of *in vitro* fertilisation.

When I first met Sonia for treatment, at the start of 2013, she had undergone three consecutive attempts to conceive and was exhausted from the experience. Towards the middle of the year, and encouraged by the possibility that her health insurance company would cover the costs of the treatment (a law had just been passed in Argentina to that effect: Law 26.862/2013. Integrated access to the procedures and medically assisted techniques of medically assisted reproduction), she decided to consult another team of professionals that had been recommended to her. She established a very good relationship with the new doctor and she felt much more support from him and from her husband, who participated more actively in the process this time. It was recommended to her that she should then consider embryo transfer.

Having undergone hormonal treatment, they were able to fertilise eight embryos, which were then frozen for future implantation. The first attempt failed as they were not able to carry out the implant. The second attempt, a short time later, similarly failed. This time, the pregnancy test was positive but, after a couple of days, she experienced an outflow and an empty sac showed up on the ultrasound.

Beyond contemplating the insistence that I saw in Sonia regarding the conception of this child, including the successive courses of treatment that she undertook (something I feel that lies close to Alkolombre's (2008) idea of the "passion for a child"), my idea here is to consider the representations that are generated in the wake of the new conception methods.

When Sonia was in the operating theatre waiting to have the embryos implanted, the doctor told her that "they are on the way" and then a lab technician appeared in his laboratory coat with "something in his hand". The scene made her think of a delivery of food.

Having carried out the procedure, the doctor approached them, gave the couple a hug and Sonia had the sensation of a "collective fertilisation". What we are considering here is not just her and her husband in the privacy of their own home—a third party is now participating in the act.

"Are the frozen embryos my children?" "Are we pregnant?" "How long?" "How is the age of the foetus calculated: from the moment of fertilisation or from the time it was implanted?" These were some of the questions that arose during sessions.

I am trying here to work through what exactly it is that has been created with these new conception methods.

Sibilia (2005) suggests that, with these planning methods for the human race, possibilities appear which belong more to the world of science fiction (today, new Golems, Frankensteins, automats, robots, and clones are possible). She asks,

> What effect do all these mutations in creation have on "modes of being"? How do we feed their construction? In other words, in what way do these transformations in context affect the processes by which what is comes into being? (Sibilia, 2008. p. 19, translated for this edition)

In the present day, the public and the private become mixed thanks to virtual reality, advances in reproductive technology have shifted the erotic dimension towards the reproductive urge, and family models are different from what was the "modern" model. We see transformations, changes in identity, and changes in the presentation of sexuality that arise out of the interaction of the body with current social norms, all dressed up in the clothing of the times. Put simply, virtual technologies exert an effect on the contemporary body and the subjectivities and ways of living space–time boundaries (Rey, 2013). We are undergoing a paradigmatic techno-scientific change.

What should we think of the new ways of making a family?

Stereotypes of the model family are today being increasingly questioned with the idea of an entity in movement and transition gaining ground all the time. Derrida and Roudinesco (2003) assert that the model Freudian family will not end up being sidelined, but do comment that it is becoming more complicated and its future is uncertain; there are many configurations which are described by the term "family" and progress in the field of genetics opens up the imagination to phenomena which are yet to be covered by civil status. In terms of law, see the contributions made by Kemelmajer de Carlucci (2011), who writes that "human assisted reproduction has created a type of intermediate category lying between biological and adoptive filiation . . . a complexity which opens up new horizons" (p. 158, translated for this edition).

Alizade (2011) also spotlights the numerous ways in which life can be brought about in the present day, based on new forms of psychosexual grouping and on new modalities of parenting: the mobility of the family constellation (the extended family), the new ways of being in a couple, the different modes of being alone. Both the human factor and psychic integrity take on an importance in terms of relevance in the exercising of healthy parenting, irrelevant of the gender of the couple. The function of the family fundamentally becomes a trophic one, including third parties who can make up for any parental deficits that exist. Here, we might think of the African proverb, "It takes the whole tribe to educate a child".

Alizade (2011) also proposes a fourth complementary series to underline "the influence exerted in the organisation of the psyche by factors originating in the sociocultural, historical, political and economic fields" (p. 75, translated for this edition). The fourth series transcends the three set out by Freud. Her intention here is to situate it at the same level as the other three and not let it be relegated to being a circumstantial factor. The imperatives of the times are being internalised and they condition thoughts and consensus on uses and customs. She believes strongly that "the apparent freedom of thought and action, the presumed authenticity of a desire, is subject . . . to the conditioning of the times . . . sociocultural contexts shape new paths" (pp. 75–76, translated for this edition).

The New Argentine Civil Code (2015) reflects this sociocultural complexity, stating that "the social reality and, in particular, family relationships are much more complex" than those encountered by Vélez Sarsfield when he drew up the Civil Code and even when Borda made a substantial overhaul of the Code in 1968, when Law 17.711 was brought into force.

Technology has transformed relationships (eggs and semen can be bought, embryos frozen, biological parents chosen, sex changed, someone donates semen to a lesbian friend, etc.).

The typical family, with mother and father as parents, seemed at one time to be set in stone. Today, we can ask, together with Alizade (2011),

> What is a family in the twenty-first century? Is living together a prerequisite for the establishing of a family? What imaginary place does it occupy in the community? What impact does the transgenerational factor have on family life? What characteristics differentiate a substitute family from a traditional one? (p. 76, translated for this edition)

The New Argentine Civil Code (2015) raises some questions on this topic.

> Many couples—of the same or different sexes—do not get married: stepfamilies, better known as "yours, mine, and ours"; single-parent

> families which come about following a decision by a woman to have a child using assisted reproduction; second or third unions in which the adults already have an economic or property framework developed and, consequently, want to choose an asset regime whereby there is no sharing of assets or "joint" assets; people with physical or mental disabilities who are allowed to get married in spite of their disability, the sharing of their life with another person being even therapeutic and beneficial to their quality of life; teenage parents who decide to bring up their child; separated partners who have a good relationship and share the care of their children after separation; individuals who, after a break-up, find themselves to be negatively affected in terms of the assets of the couple and who feel that they should be compensated for this imbalance which resulted from their giving up a career in order to look after the family home; children who have the right to take on the surnames of both parents, breaking through the sexist legal imposition of having always to adopt the surname of the father; the number of children who are now being born as a result of human assisted reproduction techniques and who are in need of clear regulations in terms of the relationships that they hold (Who are their legal parents? Who contributed the genetic material, who had the desire to procreate or the urge to be parents?); the number of children who have a right to live in, first, their own family or, this not being possible, in another family through adoption, to enumerate just some of the plethora of family realities and conflicts that contemporary society witnesses. (p. 11, translated for this edition)

Lévi-Strauss (1963[1958]) stated that "A kinship system does not consist in the objective ties of descent or consanguinity between individuals. It exists only in human consciousness; it is an arbitrary system of representations, not the spontaneous development of a real situation" (p. 50).

The family is a group that provides security for offspring and protection for adults (Ricón, 2011). There, the interest of the ego seems to predominate over the psychosexual aspects of the family and the concept of function becomes relevant. These functions include support and protection, sexual education, the learning of roles through identification, and the transmission of values. Often the environment—like a "good enough mother" (Winnicott, 1971)—fills in for the family function, making up for primary family deficiencies. The family function and the couple function designate subjectivities in a network that supports or topples the psyche.

Biological kinship today coexists alongside "outside" kinship (significant individuals intervening from "outside the family", producing relevant psychic effects which help in the structuring of the psyche). It is important here that the human comes prior to the installing of the core gender identity. Before being man or woman, the primary identification structures the being as human. We move from a binary concept to a complex one (Morin, 2009) where there are no longer universal truths, nor fixed identities. In this context, how do we perceive ourselves as parents?

Raphael-Leff (2003) suggests the term "generative identity" in thinking about how an individual is constructed psychically as a parent, independently of gender and of the subsequent choice of sexual object or sexual identity.

An online debate was held by the IPA in 2014 on the topic of new families (Puget & Nicoló Mann), allowing for an exchange on the new modalities in the construction of the family today. There, it was also suggested that dramatic social, scientific, and technological changes in recent years have allowed for new situations and modes of relating whose consequences are still far from being understood. These changes were not as a result of discoveries in psychoanalysis, but, rather, were imposed from outside. We psychoanalysts trip over them, sometimes trying to adapt in whatever way possible, while others, accepting these changes, use the bewilderment that they throw up to mould new ideas. A crisis situated in the field forced us to take into account the effects of the real world that we had previously considered as distant.

First, we must recognise the fact that being subjects of a family is not something that is a biological given. According to Puget and Nicoló Mann (2014), two criteria coexist and are superimposed. According to the first, "we are a family" due to blood links and their various metaphors, while the second tells us that the roles of parents and children are "produced": they depend on a recognition of differences and imply appropriating and inhabiting a family space through mutual respect and the necessity to do things together which are not grounded in an original debt. The parental function necessitates constant work and an amount of stability in the relationship, which will then lead to the idea of a family connected to "familiarity".

This itself implies leaving behind the idea of the family being "sacred", determined by blood ties which produce relationships for life, and starting to think of the ability of people to create roles between parents and children, ones which are not self-sufficient, but which can possibly develop, according to the circumstances. In this way, we can discover how we came to be, little by little, a family. The parental roles are continuously constructed and do not necessarily depend on the difference between the sexes or the generations. It is possible to create a family in the process of "becoming".

Faced with these new family modalities, I now propose thinking of two situations of the many that have opened up in front of us in the present day:

Unanswered questions for couples who give their consent to the cryopreservation of embryos

As Jadur and colleagues (2010) clearly state,

> the term "pre-implant embryo" is used to describe that biological material produced as a result of assisted fertilisation treatment in a laboratory using a female and a male gamete and which, according to certain scientific–biological categories, is ready to be transferred to the womb or to be cryopreserved so as to be transferred to the womb at some later stage. Once the nesting has taken place, this pre-implant embryo, or pre-embryo, becomes an implanted embryo; then, during the pregnancy, what will possibly become a future human child will develop . . . an embryo is not the same as a pre-embryo, but neither of the two, as a biological entity, is the same as the representation made of them by patients undergoing assisted fertilisation treatment. (p. 34, translated for this edition)

In the same way as each individual has a particular representation of a child, each patient has a representation of embryos which is unique (even when, as the authors point out, they have seen real images of those same embryos).

Furthermore, a legal vacuum exists in terms of what should be done and who should decide about those embryos that are not used. Who should decide what happens to them if the couple separate: the mother, the father, both, or the fertilisation centre? The destruction of embryos is not—for the moment and until legislation is enacted—carried out by fertilisation centres.

The embryo, as it holds no legal status, cannot be donated for scientific purposes, given to another couple, or destroyed. A prenatal adoption law could be one of the possible solutions for the embryos that are currently accumulating in cryopreservation units. This would allow for them to be adopted by another couple.

Sonia was informed at that time about the different options open to the couple on what to do with embryos that were not implanted. What would she have done in such a case? It is a question that she is not able to answer even today. She said that she could not have imagined donating them to another couple because she would have been left thinking of her child growing up in another family. Neither did she consider their destruction. Both possibilities are associated with abandonment. It was comforting for her to know that, in the fertilisation clinic where she had the treatment, the embryos were kept until it was decided otherwise. She now finds herself thinking about the possibility of one last attempt at pregnancy with the three pre-embryos that are still in cryopreservation. (At the time of writing this, Sonia has just had her second daughter.)

The children conceived following the donation of eggs who want to know their genetic parents

An article in *La Nación* newspaper (Buenos Aires) was titled "Identity unknown: the unexpected side of assisted fertilisation". In a video uploaded on YouTube, an adolescent who had been born using egg donation techniques explained how she was conceived: the egg of an anonymous donor and her father's sperm created the embryo which was then transferred to the womb of her mother.

In the video we can also see an aspect of assisted reproduction which has yet to be resolved in Argentina: the right of that person conceived following the donation of eggs or semen to know the identity of their biological parents. In the film *The Kids Are Alright* (Cholodenko, 2010), this topic is touched on and two of the protagonists—a girl and a boy who are each the biological child of one of two women living together and a semen donor—get to meet their biological father, while in *Chinese Puzzle* (Klapish, 2013), we can see a lesbian couple who ask a male friend (who is married and has two children) to donate sperm to conceive a child, telling him that he will not be "a conventional father".

At the present time, anonymity is guaranteed by clinics in Argentina to both donors and recipients as a way of avoiding any possible legal action related to paternity. In that way, a woman who becomes pregnant using this technique is recognised by the legal system as the mother whether or not the genetic material is hers. Today, the "procreational urge" is placed before the genetic link. The question presents itself: do any changes come about in the affective link between those children born following the donation of eggs and their parents? The right to an identity of those children runs contrary to the right of aforementioned anonymity.

Legislation in this field is moving forward: infertility is now covered under health insurance; the regulation of kinship exists concerning adoption. The new Civil Code in Argentina also establishes guidelines in terms of kinship in those cases where assisted fertilisation has been carried out, determining that the parents of the children born this way shall be deemed as those who have shown the procreational urge over and above the origin of the genetic material. Moreover, a law will be enacted to specifically regulate what happens to frozen embryos. After all, there are children who would like to have some sort of relationship with their "half brothers and sisters". (Recently, in Argentina, the state was ordered by a judge to ensure by means of legislation the preservation of donor information until such a time as there comes into force a law creating a Register of Donors.)

Once again, the question arises here concerning parenthood, both when the desire to have a child and to form a family between people who are not of the heterosexual community and also when those who have problems in conceiving naturally are involved. According to Alizade (2011), we are witnessing a "liberation of parentality" in which parenthood seems to depend more on psychic inscriptions than corporeal realities and where the human factor is placed centre stage: the need for there to be a couple with the will to be together who will be responsible for the care of the child and the symbolic transmission to that child also.

What stance, therefore, are we to take when faced with these new ways in the constitution of subjectivity? How are we supposed to think through the theme of origin?

The necessity now arises to differentiate engendering from kinship, given that engendering derives from the side of the biological substratum and the kinship—inextricably linked to transmission—

from the side of parental functions and those spaces inside the family group.

Another difference that we can spot is the distinction between the father or mother and the male or female genitor. There are two elements in the transmission, one biological and the other psychic. The genitor is the one who engenders, but the donated gamete—whether sperm or egg—is divested of its subjectivity in the moment that it becomes donated.

In the case of the children of the donor shown in the film *The Kids Are Alright* (Cholodenko, 2010), they share the genetic matter on the part of the genitor. If we are able to affirm that the mother and the father, or those who fulfil that role, are the ones who contribute the parental function of transmission of filiation, we must not forget that the genitor, male or female, is also present in parental projections and will form part of the prehistory of the subject. He or she will also play a part in the narratives of "the neurotic's family romance" (Freud, 1909c).

In the film, the donor, even when he was anonymous, occupied a place in the minds of his children. He, who had not considered the ramifications of the donation of semen in his youth, starts to consider his paternity and the desire to make a family (in fact, he starts to question his on–off relationship with another woman and what the meaning of his life was at that particular time). What the film also allows us to see is the way in which advances in the development of biotechnology and medicine and the recognition of the human rights of so-called "minorities" are transforming the idea of "parenthood" in contemporary culture, while, at the same time, throwing up different controversial perspectives on the topic.

The symbolic operations related to origins are enlarged and show themselves to be double-faceted. First, there is consanguinity: blood ties continue to have a determining value in kinship, being of great importance at a social level and having legal implications in terms of rights of filiation, while, at the same time, being of relevance in the construction of subjectivity at the level of identity. Second, filiation: of a symbolic nature, it is aware of the transmission of the psychic life and is linked to the parental urge and identificatory projects.

In the other film mentioned, *Chinese Puzzle* (Klapish, 2013), the importance of relationships between the characters and how links are constructed throughout a life is shown in diverse situations, such as when the eldest child says to his biological father that he will look after his "sister" (a girl born after the donation of semen from her biological father to a lesbian friend).

Reflections

Setting limits to technological procedures is in no way an isolated or autonomous matter. Rather, it has to do with how technology, its development and its reach, are all thought through. I feel that we should be guided neither by extreme optimism (in which man dominates nature), nor by discouraging pessimism. What we need is to reflect on the immediate effects of scientific advances, as well as the long-term ones and those which are difficult to predict.

As commonly happens, more questions are opened up concerning our day-to-day practice and, faced with this situation, we can become better informed in order to think more about, and confront, the fear of the unknown, separating fantasy and illusion from the possible and accompanying our patients on the journey to being able to achieve motherhood and construct a family.

As psychoanalysts, we commit ourselves to revealing the fears that we experience related to the changes of the times, to recognising our limitations and to allowing the debate to continue in an open manner.

Following on from the ideas presented in the IPA online debate (Puget & Nicoló Mann, 2014), it might be that we could open up to thinking of the family structure as separate from the roles of gender and centre ourselves on the attachment or connection that the child needs. New families are operating in a space without the myths and traditions that were upheld by previous generations and this implies both liberty and uncertainty. Previous generations used to tell the story of the stork to explain how a family was brought about. What story are we to tell our children today?

References

Alizade, M. (2011). Hacer la vida en el siglo XXI: familias, parejas, soledades. *Revista de la Sociedad Argentina de Psicoanálisis, 15/16*: 73–86.

Alkolombre, P. (2008). *Deseo de hijo, pasión de hijo. Esterilidad y técnicas reproductivas a la luz del psicoanálisis*. Buenos Aires: Letra Viva Editorial.

Cholodenko, L. (2010). *The Kids Are Alright*. Film. Accessed at: www.youtube.com/watch?v=muZLrR9bK0g.

Código Civil y Comercial de la Nación comentado (2015). Gustavo Caramelo; Sebastián Picasso; Marisa Herrera. – 1a edn. – Ciudad Autónoma de Buenos Aires: Infojus, v. 2.

Derrida, J., & Roudinesco, E. (2003). *De quoi demain*. París. Libraire Arthéme Fayard et Éditions Galilée.

Freud, S. (1909c). Family romances. *S. E., 19*: London: Hogarth.

Jadur, S., Duhalde, C., & Wainstein, V. (2010). Efectos emocionales de la criopreservación de embriones y su transferencia. *Revista de la Sociedad Argentina de Medicina Reproductiva, 25*(1): 33–39.

Kemelmajer de Carlucci, A. (2011). Las nuevas formas de parentalidad pensadas desde lo jurídico. *Revista de la Sociedad Argentina de Psicoanálisis, 15/16*: 157–165.

Klapish, C. (2013). *Casse-tête chinois* [Chinese Puzzle]. Film.

La Nación (2014). 18th May, 2014, Buenos Aires. Accessed at: www.lanacion.com.ar/1691804-identidad-desconocida-el-lado-no-previsto-de-la-fertilisacion-asistida.

Lévi-Strauss, C. (1963)[1958]. *Structural Anthropology*. New York. Basic Books.

Morin, E. (2009). *Introducción al pensamiento complejo*. Barcelona: Gedisa.

Puget, J., & Nicoló Mann, M. (2014). New families: what psychoanalysis has to say about them. IPA on line debate. Kimberly Kleinman. Welcome to the inaugural IPA online debate about New Families. Accessed at: www.ipa.org.uk/en/Debates/homepage_debates.aspx.

Raphael-Leff, J. (2003). Conferencia dictada sobre reproducción asistida en Buenos Aires. APdeBA.

Rey, M. A. (2013). En el terreno de lo inútil. Buenos Aires. *Revista de la Sociedad Argentina de Psicoanálisis, 17*: 189–198.

Ricón, L. (2011). Los distintos tipos de família. In: *La família suficientemente buena* (pp. 81–91). Buenos Aires: Ed. Pólemos.

Sibilia, P. (2005). *El hombre postorgánico. Cuerpo, subjetividad y tecnologías digitales*. Buenos Aires: Fondo de Cultura Económica.

Sibilia, P. (2008). *La intimidad como espectáculo*. Buenos Aires: Fondo de Cultura Económica.

Winnicott, D. W. (1971). *Playing and Reality*. London. Tavistock.

PART III

SEXUAL DIVERSITY

CHAPTER ELEVEN

Two in one: parenthood and gender in a case of intersexuality

Teresa Rocha Leite Haudenschild

In this chapter, I consider the parents' acceptance of the physical bisexuality or intersexuality of their baby, which is founded on the constitution of the psychical bisexuality of these parents. Cultural factors and scientific parameters may precipitate the designation of the baby's gender and complicate the construction of its psychical bisexuality, essential to personality development and the process of assuming a gender—a process always influenced by the designations of the parents, even if unconsciously. Psychic criteria may even surpass physical criteria, given that the aim is the harmonious psychical development of a human being, not solely in terms of sexuality. As such, even transgender options should be reconsidered from this perspective. What follows is the clinical case of Laura, aged fifty-two, who, despite having opted for the female gender, maintains her physical bisexuality.

The constitution of psychical bisexuality

Haber (1997, p. 66) states that "The bisexuality is a masculine–feminine ensemble: a psycho–corporeal–sexual 'complex' which, in principle, will become increasingly psychical, but will always maintain connections with the body" (cf. Guillaumin, 1975). The constitution of psychosexuality follows a course that begins before birth and is based on the conscious and unconscious desires and anxieties of the parents and grandparents.

Primary psychical bisexuality

After birth, in the primary relationship with the mother, based on the mother's own internalised parental couple and the realisation of this in her real life with her husband (Bion, 1987), the primary psychical bisexuality of the new-born child is constituted concomitantly with the internalisation of the psychical representations of the feminine and the masculine.

For Bion, the mother with reverie who lends her child her capacity to contain its feelings, naming them and apprehending their meanings, is a post-genital mother who has already realised the oedipal preconception and has, therefore, internalised a good couple. She has a valued place in her mind for the feminine as much as for the masculine. Bion adds that a mother with reverie must have love for the father of the child. For him, the realisations of the preconception of the thinking breast in the primary relationship, and the oedipal preconception in the secondary relationship with the parental couple, are essential to the growth of the personality.

Secondary psychical bisexuality

When a child perceives that his or her mother is looking at the father with a feminine gaze, a gaze different to the one directed at them, genital sexuality begins (Guignard, 1997). This is constructed in the way the mother lives out her own sexuality as a woman, the value she gives to the father, and her contentment with intercourse with him. This already presupposes an intergenerational transmission and the interplay of the child's own fantasies and envy. "The secondary psychical bisexuality refers to relationships with total objects, with the depressive position (Klein, 1935), and the oedipal conflict, presupposing inter and intrapsychical communication at the symbolic level" (Haudenschild, 2013, pp. 89–90).

The primary psychical bisexuality of the mother and her receptivity related to the baby's sexuality

I think that a mother with a well-constituted primary psychical bisexuality has the mental space required to receive her intersexual baby and to value it with these particular characteristics. When the baby's intersexuality is discovered early on, I believe that maternal reverie helps the baby to accept its body and assume responsibility for it.

It is in this first experience of being with the mother (Winnicott, 1949) that the child is able to be content with his or herself. What is important in this first relationship is being a human person, although undifferentiated, more than the physical sex.

The mother's desire and the designation of gender

According to Laura, her mother wanted a daughter, having been highly disappointed at having a "son" (Laura was born with a small, yet well-defined, penis). As the mother was very young—sixteen years old—she gave her baby to a maternal aunt (who later became the adoptive mother) to care for. Laura says that she had always felt that there was a secret surrounding her birth: the mother took an enormous amount of hormones during a difficult pregnancy that forced her to spend months in bed, but Laura never had the courage to ask her adoptive parents (now deceased) about her birth.

Despite having lived for a very short time with her biological parents, she often brings her biological mother (never the father) to the analysis. She describes her as being very self-centred, and relates that she always wanted her to be a girl and a "ballerina": the profession Laura went on to choose.

The secondary psychic bisexuality of the parents and their receptivity of Laura's sexuality

The first "choices" for the gender of an inter (or trans) sex child arise from the parents' secondary psychical bisexuality and the extent to which they accept their child.

I think that even prior to eighteen months, when still living with her biological mother, Laura had already perceived that her mother had a feminine gaze towards her father, which was different to the primary maternal gaze that the mother directed at her. However, I think that Laura identified with her mother's desire, wishing to be a girl to satisfy her in the hope of redirecting her mother's gaze towards her: Laura the girl. When she failed in this because the mother distanced her by giving her to the aunt and staying with the father, perhaps Laura reinforced her conviction that the only way she could avoid losing her mother was to be a girl. I believe this was an important factor in her later decision to opt for the female gender. She says she feels that if she had been a girl, her biological mother would never have given her away, would never have rejected her.

Laura in search of a place

At about eighteen months, Laura was adopted by her great aunt and uncle, at the request of her great uncle "who had always wanted a boy" because they only had one daughter who was about to leave home to marry. She describes her uncle as being very kind, yet he was completely submissive to his wife who "controlled everything" and maintained the power, criticising all members of the family, including her daughter, who, after marrying, moved into the house next door. Laura has fond memories of her stepsister who shares and comprehends her feelings of worthlessness in terms of never corresponding to their mother's expectations. Following the premature death of this older sister, Laura speaks of feeling very alone.

When she arrived to stay at her adoptive parent's house, the great aunt gave her the toys that had belonged to her stepsister, unconsciously expressing that she wanted to continue to have a girl at home. So, Laura played, and enjoyed playing, with these toys: an expression of maternal love from the aunt to her.

Laura finds a place by becoming the girl that her aunt wanted and the boy that the uncle had hoped for. Often absent due to work, he is described as being passive to his wife, and only realised that Laura was playing with girls' toys when she was already almost five, when the mothers of other children in the neighbourhood mentioned this. In response, the parents gave her a ball and took away the dolls, which Laura looks at nostalgically on top of the wardrobe. Whenever she has the opportunity to play with other girls, she does. She says to me one day at the beginning of the analysis, "Look, *My Life in Pink* (Berliner, 1997). It's me as a child . . . I also liked putting on my mother's make-up."

She describes her mother as being emotionally distant to her feelings and encouraging her to behave like a girl, highlighting her feminine traits and emphasising her femininity to the family (Haudenschild, 2003). Paradoxically, the same mother stimulated her to be a boy by saying, "pull your pipi to make it grow", and telling her that this had been the paediatrician's advice.

Given that the father had wanted a boy, he had been proud of Laura for her intelligence and performance ever since kindergarten. Once, when she was six years old, she had been asked a question by a new teacher and, when unable to answer, was subsequently ridiculed by her, which led the whole class to laugh, and Laura ran to the teacher and bit her. Her father, when called to the school, defended her. (Although I have always been referring to Laura in the feminine, as she does herself, at that time, and up to the end of high school at the age of seventeen, she used her masculine name.)

According to Laura, despite preferring her as a boy, the father did not try to impede her when she later opted to dress and act as a woman and, indeed, to live as one. However, she never chose to remove her penis, and I think that this was so that she could continue to be the boy her father had wanted. He was the one who took her to the doctor at the age of eleven when her curves began to appear: in particular her feminine bottom. "We need to help this creature!" said the doctor. Laura recalls that the two men received her with great kindness and thinks back on this as a gift. The doctor prescribes male hormones, which Laura took only once and then threw the rest of the box away.

She never menstruated and had very few body hairs during puberty, although "my voice deepened a little at this time". The family never wanted to subject her to in-depth examinations to verify that she was intersex, a fact that her body was revealing by becoming more feminine.

From the age of seventeen onwards, Laura self-administered female hormones for many years, but no longer does so today. She tells me that she went to Europe at the age of twenty-two and was obliged by the directors of her dance company to put in breast implants (hers were underdeveloped) but she took time to get used to them: "I would have stayed as I was with my little breasts". She has come for analysis because of a fear of the passing of time, of solitude: "that's why I look for friends and places where they like me . . ."

Today, Laura is fifty-two, and has had two heterosexual partners for many years, but when her last partner insisted that she removed her penis, she left him. She feels that the caresses she receives on her penis are also fundamental to "feeling her body as complete . . .". She feels she is a woman and likes to be seen and accepted as one. She is a journalist, a gifted dancer, singer, and active intellectual, writing and fighting for the acceptance of sexual diversity, and for children's rights: "they deserve a better destiny".

I believe that her choices came to be made gradually, and that she had a favourable environment in which to realise them.

Designation of gender and intersexuality

If the gender (cf. Stoller, 1968) is designated by the parents, this first designation might or might not be syntonic with the psychical constitution of the intersex child developed in the primary and secondary relationships with the parents. As I see it, if the designation of gender is constructed in the initial relationship between the psyche of the parents and of the child, then purely physical criteria must not predominate.

Martin, a three-year-old intersex boy, the mascot for a football team, has his penis removed at a renowned children's hospital in São Paulo when it is discovered that he also possesses ovaries and a uterus. This decision is made according to the criteria in place at that time (the beginning of the 1990s) which determined that internal organs should take precedence over external ones.

It is recommended to the family that they move city, change the child's name, and begin a new life.

The boy, whose gender had already been designated by the parents (who have, therefore, already received his psychosexuality at a primary and secondary level), now has to face changing his name and gender. In addition to his penis, his identity, social surroundings, and the life he was living are all amputated, too.

Beyond the parents' contribution to the psychical identity of the child, there must also be a cultural and scientific environment that is open to the child's psychosexuality and which is not based solely on physical determinants.

I think that Martin will always maintain a psychic trace of the first gender designation attributed to him by his parents, syntonic with his own psychic identity up to the age of three. The later attribution of a female identity, founded on his internal physical body, undermines three years of work in developing an identity through the psychical relationship with his parents and the environment. I also think this traumatic experience will seriously affect his psychosexual development.

Laura's psychical characteristics and gender

Laura opts for the female gender (maternal designations prevail), although she keeps the penis (as her adoptive father desired and her adoptive mother also desired unconsciously). She does not engage in ambisexual activity as is the case with transvestites, and neither does she opt definitively for the female sex as do male to female transsexuals (who choose to remove the penis and feel entirely woman, with very little conflict), and Laura's partners are long term and heterosexual.

I believe that her father's affective acceptance of her decision to be a woman made this choice less conflicting (although he really wanted her to be a boy "to continue the family" since he had only one daughter).

Family and cultural factors

In addition to the desires of the biological mother, the desires of the adoptive mother also come into play. She is described by Laura as extremely powerful: "my father, although an army officer, handed his salary over to her." This is the mother whom Laura watches dressing, putting on make-up, and giving orders to everyone. It is this mother who, enviously, criticises the size of her penis. She encourages her to be a powerful woman, yet, at the same time, orders her to stretch out her pipi. And Laura dreams about her: "I was wearing one of her dresses, grey, military, I awoke and thought: I would never wear a dress like this, it's not beautiful or feminine." A grey dress like her father's uniform, I thought to myself.

This mother appears to be a phallic mother, as described by Kafka (1992) based on Cristine Jorgensen's biography (Richards, 1983). She is a mother who maintains the omnipotent phantasy of being a man and a woman at the same time, and is able to enact this phantasy within the family, alongside a submissive, pallid man, who becomes impotent at the age of around fifty, precisely when Laura is reaching puberty. According to Laura, her stepsister, who lived next door, was criticised by the mother for giving her children too much freedom and for being too "soft" with them and with her husband.

Laura grows up amid this family madness (Richard, 1983, p. 13), receiving care from her sister, who shares her kindness with her own children and with Laura (although she, on her deathbed, tells Laura that she was very envious of her "when a boy", as the mother had preferred him and not her, as she was a woman).

To be only a woman and have surgery that would make her physically a woman was something Laura never considered. I think that remaining physically bisexual is Laura´s way of finding herself in order to feel "powerful" enough to be valued as a person (according to the model presented by her mother–aunt).

Being a woman and having heterosexual male partners, as Laura did, is to be the woman her biological mother wanted her to be, while also being a woman like her caring sister. Keeping her penis also means identifying with the caring men who looked after her: her adoptive and biological fathers, the latter being described in the most recent sessions of analysis as being very caring and not at all submissive to his wife, unlike the adoptive father: he was a rebel, like the men in *Rebel Without A Cause* (Ray, 1955), always with his motorbike. If he did not like the atmosphere, he left.

This father's attitude is a counterpoint to Laura's terror of "not having a place". He was sure he was able to leave and then come back and that his place was guaranteed alongside Laura's mother. He stayed with her mother while Laura was sent out of the house to live in the house of the aunt–mother, where she would have to search for a place either as daughter-of-the-mother (aunt) or as her phallic extension (as a boy).

I think that Laura held on to a rebellious trace of the father, who brought her up by not accepting surrounding impositions; however, although his rebelliousness is to simply flee the situation, Laura's is primarily to stop and think and see what is best for her.

Today, after more than fifty years, Laura has rekindled the relationship with her biological family, having spent the last Christmas with them, searching for her place there, among her very caring sisters. She recounts that every time she phoned, her mother would unleash an avalanche of complaints, and a list of illnesses. Laura would listen to her and afterwards her affectionate father would ask, "When are you coming to see us? It's a joy when you are here." Laura is happy to be received this way by him, as she was before by her adoptive father.

Laura's analysis

The fears of not being welcome were, as I understand it, those that drove Laura to come for analysis when she returned to her initial parental home. The "anguish of not having a place" has always been within her, and at times when everyday life presents an unfavourable situation in this sense, she relives this anguish with great intensity. During one carnival, while performing as a late and celebrated Brazilian musician, she is complimented effusively by a journalist, but tells me that "when he discovered that I was not *only* a woman, he passed the microphone to the director of the samba school, not giving me an opportunity to say anything. He didn't give me a voice . . . And as I have been through this a lot, I will always fight for those who don't have a voice."

Laura comes for analysis to "give voice" to these buried (Freud, 1937d) primitive anxieties, related to the feeling that ever since birth she never had a place with her mother where she could exist in her individuality.

The analysis opens the way to making sense of primary initial experiences, which, in her case, had never been lived through, because there was no experience of being at one with a mother who named her anxieties and desires. In this sense, the neo-sexualities are more closely related to a basic failure in the feeling of narcissistic continuity, as in borderline cases, than to psychosis or perversion (cf. Chiland, 2000, 2005).

It also opens up the possibility of re-elaboration of later secondary affective oedipal experiences, integrating these with primary experiences.

While there is "the danger of an attempt by the patient to adapt to what the analyst or culture supposes is healthier or more correct" (Marucco, 2007), the work of analysis is not that of "offering adaptations or reconstructing fragments of a past history", but, rather, of "constructing in the transferential present what is lacking in the story, establishing a liberation diachronically in the analysis" unique to each analysand. In the moment that Laura "gives voice" to the anguish related to her bodily constitution, she may become more "free" to think something that, for the family, was "unthinkable". The analysis continues unfolding, with my listening (Haudenschild, 2013) as freely as is possible, to hear her living psychic singularity.

Acknowledgement

I am grateful to Christopher Mack for his work as translator.

References

Berliner, A. (1997). *Ma vie en rose* (Film). Haut & Court, WFE, Freeway Films.

Bion, W. R. (1987). *A Theory of Thinking. Second Thoughts*. London: Karnac.

Chiland, C. (2000). The psychoanalyst and the transsexual patient. *International Journal of Psychoanalysis, 81*: 21–35.

Chiland, C. (2005). Problèmes posés aux psychanalystes par les transsexuels. *Revue française de psychanalyse, 69*(2), 563–577.

Freud, S. (1937d). Constructions in analysis. *S. E., 23*: 257–269. London: Hogarth.

Guignard, F. (1997). *Le sourire du chat. Epître à l'objet*. Paris: PUF.

Guillaumin, J. (1975). Bisexualité vécue et bisexualité rêvée. *Revue française de psychanalyse, 39*: 893–704.

Haber, M. (1997). Identité, bisexualité psychique et narcissisme. *Bissexualité – Monographies de la Revue Française de Psychanalyse*, 49–67.

Haudenschild, T. (2003). *The Green Continent: The Constitution of Femininity in a Clinical Case. Studies on Femininity*. London: Karnac.

Haudenschild, T. (2013). Listening to psychical bisexuality in analysis. In: E. Palerm & F. Thomson-Salo (Eds.), *Masculinity and Femininity Today* (pp. 87–100). London: Karnac.

Kafka, E. (1992). The influence of the parents' unconscious fantasies on children's adaptation as illustrated by transsexuality. *Journal of Clinical Psychoanalysis, 1*: 547–559.

Klein, M. (1935). A contribution to the psychogenesis of manic–depressive states. *International Journal of Psychoanalysis, 16*: 145–174.

Marucco, N. (2007). Between the remembering and the destiny: the repetition. Presented to the IPA International Congress, Berlin.

Ray, N. (1955). *Rebel Without a Cause* (Film). Warner.

Richards, R. (1983). *Second Serve*. New York: Stein & Day.

Stoller, R. (1968). *Sex and Gender (Volume 1)*. New York: Science House.

Winnicott, D. W. (1949). *The Ordinary Devoted Mother and Her Baby*. Private publication.

CHAPTER TWELVE

The neuter gender and the setting up of psychosexuality

Ana Maria Rocca Rivarola

The setting-up of psychosexuality can be seen as the way that a person integrates their body and genital perception, their erotic sexuality, their conscious and unconscious fantasies, their experiences and their identification with their first objects. All of this contributes towards building a feeling about themselves as a sole group of masculine and feminine elements that define the way in which each person will place him or herself in the world and relate with the others.

The development of the biological sexuality, from conception to puberty, occurs in a discontinuous and differentiated process where a series of transformations in different aspects (chromosomal, gonadal, hormonal, and genital) occurs. However, there are other change factors in the human being that overlap with biological development and which are in the origin of the setting up of the psychosexuality and which intervene favouring or hindering its evolution. Some of these factors are:

1. The way that the child's sex is perceived by the parents (and by the environment) depends on their desires and expectations (conscious and unconscious) and which expresses itself since birth in the mother–child relationship.

2. The pre-oedipal attachment or the initial identification of the child with the mother. The meeting with this first object is what will define the type of psychic structuring that is not based on the recognition of the other marked by personal and sexual difference, but on a type of undifferentiated bond, where the other is seen as neuter and as a part of themselves (narcissism).
3. The child's identification with the masculine and feminine aspects of the father and the mother. The articulation of this identification will determine the child's feeling of belonging to the masculine or feminine gender.
4. The presence of the father in the mother's mind and in the child's mind, as well as his or her real physical presence, will allow the child to leave the symbiotic relationship with the pre-oedipal mother and to establish bonds that relate her individually to the mother and the father, while, at the same time, confronts her with the existing bond between the parents in which the child does not participate, but is a witness to this. This makes it possible for the child to perceive himself as a separate person from the mother and to relate with others, passing thus from bi-dimensionality (where the perception of the object does not exist) to tri-dimensionality (where the perception of the object and the separation exists). The subject is conscious of the discontinuity of the presence of the object, and its occasional unavailability and, therefore the existence of other objects and the possibility of relating to them recognising the difference and the incompleteness that cause the pain of separation and makes the subject perceive the importance of desire for both the object and him or herself (the oedipal triangular conflict).

Green (1983) in his paper "The neuter gender" (Le genre neutre) suggests that certain psychopathological structures seem to be set in a period of time where there is no sexual differentiation. In these cases, the subject feels he is neither a man nor a woman. Any hetero- or homosexual aspiration is eliminated from their behaviour and their desire. This neuter gender fantasy, built up with the resources of a predominant narcissism, bears the markings of a megalomaniac ideal ego. In fact, in terms of desire, the vision is either all or nothing: "As I can't have everything or be everything, I will have and be nothing". The child builds up this fantasy based on the perception of the maternal fantasy that desires that the son/daughter have neither a sex nor be alive. The neuter gender fantasy appears as a manifestation of obedience towards the mother's desire and, at the same time, as a way of getting revenge on her by violent rejection (Green, 1983, p. 208).

Freud in his article "Female sexuality", states that in this child's dependence on the mother we have the origin of later paranoia in women. For it appears that this origin is the surprising, yet regular, dread of being killed (devoured) by the mother. It would seem plausible to conjecture that this anxiety corresponds to the hostility which the child develops towards her mother because of the manifold restrictions imposed by the latter in the process of training and physical care and that the immaturity of the child's psychical organisation favours the mechanism of projection (Freud, 1931b, p. 520).

The father's presence allows the passage from the mother's lap to the father's, allowing the child to perceive himself as an individual, separated from the mother, and with the possibility of relating with others, enlarging the possibilities of containment and the flow of feelings of love and hate. If the father is absent, the pre-eminence of the pre-oedipal attachment with the mother would persist, where the only possibility is to establish an undifferentiated and asexual dyadic relationship.

Along the path that the woman travels from her birth to motherhood, she relives her initial identification with her mother and her father. During the transformation of motherhood, the triangular scene that created the child can became "dual" if the mother abandons her feminine position (as the man's companion) and seeks refuge with the child (or through the child) in a symbiotic relationship, an undifferentiated one that excludes sexuality (in terms of the recognition of the female–male differentiation). In this case, the baby, facing the threat of not being, does not have any other option except to be the "mother's unfulfilled desire". In this situation, the dynamics of the woman–mother's sexual desire towards her partner will be fundamental to reinstall the oedipal triangle which is capable of placing a limit on undifferentiated symbiosis. The father should not only be present in the desire and the mother's mind, his active presence is also important as a father and as the mother's companion. He should also renounce the tendency to place himself as a "son" in the relationship with the woman (now transformed into a mother) in an attempt to revive the symbiotic link with his own mother, in order to take on the masculine position of a man who, with his desire, demands that the woman take up the female position. In this way, he will prevent the woman from being tied to a symbiotic link with the child, allowing the transformation of maternal to female.

The sexualisation that creates the Oedipus complex, where there is the recognition of the other, of the sexual differentiation and of the incompleteness, breaks the spell of the neuter, of the asexual, the narcissistic, that, in serious situations, provokes near sinister feelings (Marucco, 2012).

The masculine and feminine sexual desire of the mother and the father allows the oedipal triangle to be recovered. Thus, the baby is saved from the symbiotic relationship with the pre-oedipal mother and the mother is saved from the symbiotic relationship with the child.

When the mother has a well-structured psychic bisexuality with a good parental internalisation from the relationship with each one of her parents, she can offer the baby a gaze that accepts him or her in their individuality from their birth (Haudenschild, 2009, p. 123).

The lack of an internal-object father, who is firmly installed in the mother's unconscious oedipal object relationship, creates an emotional vacuum that removes an essential gradient for the psychological impersonal elaboration of the oedipal triangle (Ogden, 1992). In this case, the function of the analysis is to allow the patient to recover from the undifferentiated, from the tendency towards psychic death. The position of the analyst is fundamental because their posture of man/woman that recognises the difference, the feminine and masculine that characterises them, will allow the patient to reach, in their psychic life, the recognition of separation, of incompleteness, of the other, of the masculine, and of the feminine. Thus, the analytic work opens the opportunity for the patients to construct themselves as individuals finding, as much as they possibly can, their own way to live their sexuality, to develop their thinking capacity, to creatively transform reality, and to relate with others, making them the authors of their own lives.

Clinical material

Moira is currently thirty-two years old. She is a very skilled medical doctor. She is an only child who was born with a genetic malformation syndrome that presents different characteristics: her hands are deformed; at birth she had cleft palate (which was operated on when she was a small child); she does not have much hair, has baby teeth, and is very thin and short. Her physical appearance is hybrid and fragile. She dresses in an undifferentiated manner, wearing only trousers and neutral colours. The genetic malformation does not affect the genital organs, yet she had a blurring sexuality that is related to how she constituted her identity. The state of physical vulnerability arising from this malformation had an influence on the type of symbiotic relationship that Moira has had with her mother, which was reinforced by the absence of the father (who remained emotionally distant from the patient until she was thirteen years old, and after this age was completely absent, as he died in an accident).

Moira's condition prevented her from developing emotionally and sexually, although intellectually she has had a good development. A clear split in her personality can be observed. As a medical doctor, she is very knowledgeable; however, affectively she remained in an extreme childlike state. Over several years of analysis, she evolved from a state in which she felt practically a baby (at the time she began her analysis, she was in her third year of medical school, and the mother fed her by mouth) to the current situation in which she is trying to differentiate herself from the mother and build her own identity. Her interaction with others outside the work environment is very poor. She hardly speaks to men, only connecting with them professionally. In her world, men are distant and unknown. She lives surrounded by women (relatives and co-workers) and has no friends except for a gay friend, with whom she makes unsuccessful attempts to imagine herself as a woman in a relationship with a man.

According to Moira, her parents had a cold and distant relationship. She was never able to see them as a couple. She was very jealous of her father, considered him a rival, and wished that he would die, so that she could be alone with her mother. When her father died, Moira had the omnipotent feeling that she had managed to kill him with her wish. After the father's death, Moira started sleeping in her mother's bed.

She went to college in a city close to her home town. In the first year of analysis, she travelled back and forth every day to her mother's house. Later, she bought an apartment and settled in the city where she studied and now works at the university. Moira's mother visits her every week, during which she cleans the house, cooks, and washes Moira's clothes. During the analysis, Moira has gradually been able to achieve some changes. First, she was able to leave her mother's bed and sleep in another bed in the same room, and then she got a room to herself. Despite the difficulties, which, at the beginning of the analysis, seemed insurmountable, she graduated from medical school and did her residency, including the third year of her residency in a city far from her home town and an internship for a few months abroad. Slowly, she has been able to detach herself from her mother, at least physically, and work actively in her analysis to differentiate herself from other people and find her place as an individual.

Moira's analysis

Moira began her analysis over ten years ago. Currently, she has sessions three times a week. At the time she began analysis, she was twenty-two years old and in the third year of medical school. The reason that led her to seek help was that she felt incapable of continuing her studies. She was very distressed, physically and mentally weakened. She found it difficult to interact with colleagues from school, and she could not attend meetings or parties. Social events produced unbearable anguish that caused her to feel dizzy. When attending conferences, she often became sick, and could not eat in public because she would often vomit. She regularly had a cold.

For Moira, the work done in analysis was like a second birth, in the sense of the attempt to construct aspects of her identity that she had never developed before. During the many years of analysis, she built a more consistent feeling about herself, beginning to imagine herself separate from others. She somatises less, and can reflect on her undefined and neuter position and own a desire for differentiation, trying to find her own way to be herself and live her sexuality.

Sometimes, she gets depressed as, at thirty-two, she thinks it is too late and not possible, but at other times she can feel and express the wish to discover something true about herself, something that gives meaning to her life. For example, at the end of a recent session, she said, "It is suffering [referring to her malformation] but this is my life, either I have this or I die. It is worth it because it is this that I have to live. I feel like living to know new things, to elaborate everything that is unresolved in my life."

Moira has lately brought many dreams to analysis, which, in my view, show her hard inner work to take hold of herself as well as the dynamics of her analysis.

> In the analytical situation, dreams can change, they can be communications for the analyst, gifts, courtesy acts for the analyst and elaboration process expressions as an answer to the analyst`s interpretation. In this way, the dreams also reflect what is happening in the analyst–patient relationship in terms of transference. (Rocha Barros, 2011, p. 45, translated for this edition)

The analyst has always to be very attentive to perceive and discriminate when Moira's movements and dreams are attempts to establish a symbiotic relationship with her, in tune with what she imagines the analyst's wish is, and when they are the true expressions of the working through process as an answer to the analyst's interpretation.

Let me illustrate, with some of Moira's dreams, moments of this analysis.

Vignette 1

Moira: I had a dream. There was a church and there was a copy of this church in another place and, at a certain point it was as if they were stuck together: one that was old and the other that was new. The old one was to be demolished because there was no reason to keep it, but afterwards, when they were side by side, I think that if the old one were demolished this could ruin the other.

When I woke up I remembered the dream, but later it disappeared, as if suddenly my mind sank and the memory of the dream was lost.

Comment

The "church" in this dream, in my opinion, represents the internal organisation that guards the sacred, Moira's essence that is entangled with her mother. Moira expresses here the perception of the necessity to separate herself from this undifferentiated relationship to be able to find her own boundaries, her own identity, but, at the same time, shows her how separation is felt to be a threat of destruction of both the self and the object.

Vignette 2

Moira: I dreamed that I was in Peru about to come back to Brazil and I wanted to walk on the street, but it was dangerous, I could be robbed; suddenly various people could come and take things from me. Although I knew it was dangerous, I decided to go out to get to know the place. I had a sensation of immunity; nothing would happen to me. And, in fact, four boys came and grabbed my arms and legs and wanted to take my handbag. I asked them to let me get my documents because I couldn't return to Brazil without them. I show them my hands (something I never do) as if saying: "Don't you feel sorry for me?" In the end, I don't know if they took my handbag; they left, I don't know if they took something. When I was alone again, I felt like walking on the street, but I had lost the sensation of immunity. The worst thing for me was not getting to know the city. This sensation of immunity was as if I was a special person, protected. Then I discovered I am just an ordinary person: I am not special, I am not different.

When I am robbed I show my hands as if I wanted to take advantage of this to protect myself. But it is very aggressive, four people pulling at me! How could I fight against four men?! There is no way. In my dream, I felt sorry for myself. I use this showing of my hands to get out of the situation. I don't feel sorry for myself. As I'm not strong, either I do this through strength or through fragility.

I didn't want to stay in Peru but I don't know if this place was bad. If they had stolen my documents, I would not have the option to live or to stay; without documents I wouldn't have any choice. I think that many times in life, each one makes their choices. Some choices are so difficult that we feel that there is no choice. A colleague who is a professor says that I have to become a professor, that I have the profile of a professor. On the one hand, I feel flattered, on the other, I think this does not have to be good for her, it has to be good for me.

Analyst Maybe Peru [in Portuguese, "Peru" is a euphemism for the male sexual organ] represents masculine sexuality that you live very aggressively and think that if you face this you would lose your identity (your documents). The handbag could represent your femininity, your sexuality that could be stolen, taken by force by the masculine aggressive sexuality.

You also don't know if feeling like a woman in front of a man is good or not, you are afraid, you still think that you prefer to go back to this conception of yourself with which you are already identified: going back to Brazil would be like a Moira who does not face masculine sexuality (Peru) and does not need to position herself as a woman.

[Moira agrees and becomes thoughtful.]

Analyst: This reminds me of the previous session. When you spoke about the film, *Departures*, it seems as if you left out a part in your description . . .

Moira: [laughs] A part of the film that I left out . . . I don't know what I said and what I didn't say.

Analyst: What happens when the main character prepares the body of the person that died?

Moira: Oh! Yes! The first body that he prepares seems to be the body of a woman but then he realises that it is a man. In the end, the important thing is the dead person's choice. The body is prepared just as the person had chosen to live; it is prepared as a woman. There is acceptance by the father, the family . . . [She becomes thoughtful] How can you separate the thoughts that belong to another person from those that are really mine?

When John [a homosexual friend] said, "To me you are a man in a woman's body", I wanted to beat him up. I wanted him to see me as a woman.

Analyst: Neither of you was accepting the other one. You didn't want to accept that he was a homosexual and wanted him to look at you "as a man looks at a woman". And he didn't want to accept you as a woman.

Moira: I had another dream. I was in the bathroom and a woman comes in and touches my bottom as if she were picking me up. I'm surprised and think, what should I do now? I become paralysed. My feeling was ambiguous and I asked myself, "Why don't you get close to her to see what happens?" But I don't do this; I end up leaving and going away.

Analyst: Now you are talking about another vision that sees you as a homosexual object. It seems as if you, here in your analysis, are trying to find yourself, define who you are, discover your sexuality. You realised that you don't want to be seen (or see yourself) as if you were a man (John's vision) and you also don't want to be seen (or see yourself) as a homosexual (the woman in the dream).

Moira: In this sense, John is better defined than me: he feels like a man and likes men. I wanted to feel like a woman, but I don't feel capable. I cannot get close to a man, I don't even know what a man is like; they are so distant that they are not part of my life. I cannot die because I feel so incomplete that if I died now, it would seem that my life had no meaning, as if I left out experiencing something very important. Something very essential is missing; without this, it seems that the rest does not hold up. This is the reason why I'm so attached to my profession.

Analyst: How can you express something that you feel is missing?

Moira: I want to feel like a woman, break this barrier, this shell that leaves my femininity so suffocated, I cannot give it a format, I don't know how. I feel I'm nothing. If I were the body in the film [*Departures*], I wouldn't be able to say anything; they could only say, "Do not fix her hair, don't put on anything, no colour, put on white clothing, because this person didn't manage to be anything, she is undifferentiated."

Analyst: You are trying to find your own colours here, your way to feel alive and be yourself.

Comment

In her first dream, Moira is in Peru, as if she is a masculine organ, wanting to know the world of sexuality of man, of the other who is different, but feels that it is dangerous to show herself. Wanting to know this world is very threatening. This trip also seems to be the analysis, a dangerous trip leading to the discovery of herself. She discovers that she is not immune to pain which means she perceives her fragility, her incompleteness, the shock of what is different, the masculine, which is felt to be threatening and aggressive. She wants to protect herself from this exposure to sexuality, supporting herself on the image she has of herself that she is used to: she shows herself to be a disabled and fragile person. She shows the deformity in her hands so that people pity her. During her analysis, she feels pain when she perceives that I, her analyst, can be on her side, but I am not inside her, we are two separate people.

Her mother's attitude to Moira is similar to that of the woman in the second dream, who touches her, picking her up, as if she were a "homo object" mummy's boy, or the mother's phallus. In her fantasy, the mother's position is confused. Maybe she would have preferred her to have been a boy.

She imagines genital sexuality as something violent and invasive; it is a fight where they can take her femininity (her bag) and her identity (her documents) away from her. She has the fantasy of an aggressive primal scene. She cannot have a sexual relationship; she cannot betray her mother with a man as her mother gave up sex for her.

She can develop professionally because it is an area with fewer conflicts; she has a professional identity that, despite being partial, is something that gives her autonomy. From this, she can develop other aspects of herself and can try to get out of the symbiotic link with her mother.

In the session, we could highlight the importance of the other's perception of her in the definition of her identity.

When she comments on the film, *Departures*, she talks about the importance of the other's acceptance to be able to define the sexual identity of the "dead body". In the dream, if she were seen as a woman, she would be raped, so she tries to be perceived as a fragile and disabled person in order to be spared.

There is also the perception of the homosexual friend who cannot see her as a woman. The woman of the second dream seems to represent the mother's perception, which sees her as a homosexual object, Dora's perception that expects something from her professional postion.

Finally, there is the analyst's perception that intends to be a comprehensive one to allow her to develop, find her own individuality, and define the way to feel and live her sexuality.

Vignette 3

Moira: I dreamed I was in your house; it was in the morning. You were with your husband in the kitchen and I try to come in to have breakfast, but when I open the door, you get angry with me and say, "No, you can't come in here!" and close the door. I'm very hurt and, at the same time, curious: why don't you let me in?

Comment

In this dream, Moira expressed, on the one hand, the desire to be within the "home-mind" of the analyst, in a link in which there is no separation. At the same time, she begins to perceive the other as a separate person. The consequence of this is the discovery that she and her mother–analyst–object are not alone in the world, that the object relates to another that is not Moira (baby): it is the third element that symbolises the father. This would mark the transition from bi-dimensionality to tri-dimensionality. Thereafter, Moira begins to imagine and fantasise about the secret relationship between two partners who, in fact, exclude her in order to enjoy mutually an intimate relationship. The consciousness of the discontinuity of the object's presence, its occasional unavailability, and, therefore, the existence of other objects, makes her feel the pain of separation and realise the importance of the desire for both the object and herself.

Some conclusions

Although Moira is chronologically an adult, in her analysis we are constantly focusing on child and adolescent aspects and the patient develops aspects that were never built before. As in the case of an adolescent, who is in a full development process, Moira's analysis also serves to open up the opportunity for building aspects of herself that are potentially present, but they have no form and are not fully defined.

The patient and the analyst had to live and overcome a sense of dismay in the transference–countertransference, the feeling that it was not worth investing in the analysis because Moira felt too limited to develop as a person. To the extent that the analyst can invest in the analysis, overcoming that feeling, Moira responds, collaborating actively with a rich production of dreams. Dreams are images from which thoughts and words come, to form deep and diffuse feelings that have no known words and thoughts, and when they are thought in "the here and now" of the transference, they can be transformed to halt the trend towards nothing, to neuter, to death, which often dominates the patient. So, through analytic work, Moira can gradually accept her limitations and realise her possibilities, finding her own way to be herself and to live her sexuality.

As Green says (1995),

> We could ask ourselves: What is important? What has more value? Life's value is linked to what all human beings share and aspire: the need to love, to enjoy life, to be part of a relationship in its fullest expression, etc. Once again we find ourselves confronted with our ideology in regard to what psychoanalysis is good for. What would be its goal? Overcoming our primitive anxieties? Repairing our objects damaged by our badness? Meeting the need for security? Following adaptation standards? Or be able to feel alive and invest in the many possibilities offered by the diversity of life, despite the inevitable disappointments, sources of unhappiness and burden of suffering? (Green, 1995, p. 878)

McDougall, in her book *The Many Faces of Eros*, writes,

> If societies seek to safeguard social survival and medicine seeks to protect biological survival, could not psychoanalysis declare as its goal to safeguard the factors contributing to the psychic survival of human beings? But what is 'psychic survival', exactly? Perhaps it could be defined as the individual's ability to sustain a sense of identity in its dimensions both subjective and sexual, as well as to maintain a sense of narcissistic stability, even though the self-esteem levels are constantly affected by fluctuating conditions. (1995, p. 256)

References

Freud, S. (1931b). Female sexuality. *S. E., 21*: 225–243. London: Hogarth.

Green, A. (1983). Le gendre neutre. In: *Narcissisme de vie, narcissisme de mort* (pp. 231–245). Paris: Éditions de Minuit.

Green, A. (1995). Has sexuality anything to do with psychoanalysis? *International Journal of Psychoanalysis, 76*(5): 871–883.

Haudenschild, T. (2009). O pai e a constituição da masculinidade. *Jornal de Psicanálise, 77*: 123–141.

Marucco, N. (2012). Lo Arcaico y lo Femenino-Masculino, Metapsicologia, clínica y técnica. Paper presented to Congresso Latino-americano de Psicanálise (FEPAL), São Paulo.

McDougall, J. (1995). *The Many Faces of Eros: A Psychoanalytic Exploration of Human Sexuality*. New York: W. W. Norton.

Ogden, T. (1992). The threshold of the male Oedipus complex. In: *The Primitive Edge of Experience* (pp. 141–186). London: Karnac.

Rocha Barros, E. (2011). Sonhos. *Revista Brasileira de Psicanálise, 45*(2): 45.

CHAPTER THIRTEEN

Countertransference in psychodynamic psychotherapy of gender identity disorder patients

Cláudio Laks Eizirik, Stefania Pigatto Teche, and Guilherme Kirsten Barbisan

In this chapter we discuss the definition and history of the concept of gender dysphoria currently described as gender identity disorder. The countertransference involved in the process of analytic psychotherapy and evaluation for the sex reassignment surgery is examined. The feelings aroused in this process must be acknowledged and worked on so they are not restricted merely to enactments and resistances. Clinical illustrations featuring relevant topics for the treatment of gender dysphoria patients in psychodynamic psychotherapy are discussed. The topic shows the sexual diversity increasingly found in psychotherapy and analysis.

Introduction

In conjunction with our contemporary culture, psychoanalysis has been challenged to understand the new family settings and a broad sexual diversity, as well as to handle new clinical situations and patients and families showing new psychopathologies and relationships. Among them, gender dysphoria has been extensively studied to understand biological, psychological, and behavioural mechanisms that explain this phenomenon. The area of sex and gender is highly controversial and has led to a proliferation of terms whose meanings vary over time and within and between disciplines, as we can see from the names given over the years by the different psychiatric diagnostic manuals such as the *DSM* and *ICD* to define dysphoria gender. An additional source of confusion is that in English, "sex" connotes both male and female and sexuality.

The term transsexual emerged in the professional literature based on Hirschfeld's writings in 1923. Nevertheless, it was only in 1940 that it took on a connotation similar to its current one: individuals wishing to live, or in fact living, permanently in the opposite social role of their assigned gender and who wanted to have sex reassignment surgery. In 1973, Fisk proposed the term "gender dysphoria syndrome" which was meant to include transsexuality and all other gender identity disorders.

The 1992 *International Classification of Diseases-10* (WHO, 1992) provides five different possible diagnoses for the gender identity disorders. The term gender dysphoria shows up for the first time as a diagnosis in the fifth issue of the *DSM*. The current term sees the dysphoria as a clinical problem instead as one's own identity. According to the *DSM-5* (American Psychiatric Association, 2013), gender dysphoria as a general descriptive term refers to an individual's affective/cognitive discontent with the assigned gender. Gender dysphoria, when used as a diagnostic category, refers to the distress that might accompany the incongruence between one's experienced or expressed gender and one's assigned gender. Gender identity is a category of social identity (which usually corresponds to a person's anatomical sex) and refers to an individual's identification as male, female, or, occasionally, some category other than male or female, and gender assignment refers to one's natal assignment as a man or a woman. Transgender refers to the broad spectrum of individuals who transiently or persistently identify with a gender different from their natal gender. Transsexual denotes an individual who seeks, or has undergone, a social transition from male to female or female to male, which in many, but not all, cases also involves a somatic transition by cross-sex hormone treatment and genital surgery (sex reassignment surgery).

The *DSM-5* defines only four possible diagnoses: (1) gender dysphoria in children; (2) gender dysphoria in adolescents and adults;

(3) other specified gender dysphoria (duration less than six months); (4) unspecified gender dysphoria. The manual (*DSM-5*) lists the main characteristics of gender dysphoria (in adults and adolescents) as: (a) a marked incongruence between one's experienced/expressed gender and assigned gender, of at least six months' duration; (b) a strong desire to be rid of one's primary and/or secondary sex characteristics; (c) a strong desire for the primary and/or secondary sex characteristics of the other gender; (d) a strong desire to be of the other gender (or some alternative gender different from one's assigned gender); (e) a strong desire to be treated as the other gender (or some alternative gender different from one's assigned gender); (f) a strong conviction that one has the typical feelings and reactions of the other gender (or some alternative gender different from one's assigned gender).

Although some authors maintain the idea that there is a group of pure transsexual patients for whom the surgery would be strongly recommended, the fact is that gender dysphoria manifests itself differently in different groups and the patients who wish for gender reassignment surgery are part of a diverse group of individuals suffering from a wide range of disorders (Ruiz et al., 2014).

The gender dysphoria phenomenon is not explained by a one-size-fits-all theory. Studies have shown several clinical variants for these patients, including stigmatised homosexuals, sadists, masochists, eonists, borderlines, and transvestites. Lothstein (1977a) says that, despite presenting a vast array of psychiatric disorders, in his experience patients show points in common, such as a tendency to use primitive defence mechanisms, a constellation of obsessive and schizoid traits, and a potential to decompensate under stress in a psychotic manner. Psychological test results from gender dysphoria and long-term psychotherapy patients showed a prevalence of borderline disorders, latent schizophrenia, and an impulsive paranoid character. Most patients have a history of inadequate maternal care and debilitated object relationships. In his work with 125 patients seeking surgery, Lothstein (1977b) believes that in a small number of patients, the transsexualism could be explained by neurological, hormonal, and biological aetiologies, and suggests there is an important maternal contribution to the patients' gender disorders.

Given the possibility of undergoing sex-changing surgery, many patients have searched for healthcare services for that purpose. They are submitted to clinical, hormonal, psychiatric, and psychological evaluations, and are offered psychotherapy to handle this process. Each patient discusses their own history during psychotherapy. However, common characteristics have been detected in the course of these patients' analytic psychotherapy. One of the challenges faced by therapists during the psychotherapy of gender dysphoria patients is to manage countertransference. In the course of treatment, these cases arouse very intense feelings, such as anger, fear, confusion, and, frequently, a sense of powerlessness and passivity.

In the case illustrated throughout the chapter, the therapist was feeling mostly confused and finding it hard to have a therapeutic relationship with the patient. By understanding the case with the supervisors, the countertransference was better understood, the therapist became less confused, and therapeutic relationship became more significant.

Countertransference

Countertransference represents a set of the therapist's unconscious manifestations related to his/her patient's transference. These manifestations are part of the analytic field developed by the therapist–patient dyad and serve as a work tool capable of assessing empathy and guiding interpretations. Countertransference might compromise the treatment if it is not identified (Eizirik & Lewkowicz, 2014).

As knowledge and use of countertransference has advanced, countertransference has become one of the fundamental concepts for the practice of psychoanalysis and analytical psychotherapy. This concept was introduced by Freud (1910d) in his work, "The future prospects of psycho-analytic therapy". However, he published very little about the topic and mostly highlighted its negative influence on the treatment process from the standpoint that such influence derives from the physician's internal complexes and resistances, which should be dealt with via self-analysis. Hence, Freud believes countertransference is an obstacle to analysis that must be overcome by the analyst.

Although Freud (1912e) considered countertransference an obstacle to treatment, when he refers to hovering attention he describes how the physician's unconscious may be used as a "therapeutic tool", something later confirmed by subsequent findings.

Etchegoyen (1987) notes that the forty years between Freud's discovery of countertransference and the time its studies resume cannot be said to have gone by in vain. However, it is certain they did not bring anything substantially new about the topic. He highlights studies by Theodor Reik and Fenichel where they outline a theory of countertransference based on intuition, although they did not formulate it.

From the late 1940s and early 1950s, countless studies emerged that led to a new concept of totalistic countertransference. Many of those studies were conducted based on the analysis of more disturbed patients that evoked more intense countertransference reactions.

Heimann's (1950) "On countertransference" is the work regarded as the turning point for the countertransference concept. In it, the author uses the term countertransference to describe all of the reactions an analyst experiences towards a patient. Racker had put forward similar ideas a few years before. However, Heimann was the first to publish internationally. Etchegoyen (1987) emphasises that Racker's studies are more systematic and complete. Additionally, he published a series of papers, unlike Heimann who published only two articles on the topic in 1950 and another ten years later.

From these developments, our understanding about countertransference followed different pathways. On the one hand, in the USA, the so-called classic concept prevailed, while the totalistic concept was prevalent in Latin America and England.

From the classic concept, countertransference is restricted to the analyst's unconscious reaction to the patient's transference. It is not considered a regular element in the analytic situation but rather as something solely disruptive. Some authors also believe that expanding the countertransference concept might take the therapist away from his/her ideal position of neutrality.

The totalistic concept considers countertransference a normal phenomenon in the therapeutic process. Kernberg (1965) further posits that, when the therapist uses his/her emotional reactions to understand the patient, he/she ends up with greater freedom to observe the patient's feelings. Starting in the 1970s, the totalistic concept gained momentum and began increasingly influencing the authors of the classic countertransference model. This movement seems to derive from findings about the importance of countertransference in psychoanalytic studies of deeply disturbed children and patients (borderlines and psychotics), among which studies Kernberg's stands out.

The totalistic concept started being criticised as well, despite its progress, for failing to tell apart that which comes from the analyst and that which comes from the patient. Sandler and colleagues (1970) emphasise the risk that the concept might become a "hodgepodge" mixed up with the therapist's psychological reality. Hence, these warnings led to the consideration that there may be two sources producing the therapist's emotional manifestations in the course of a session: his/her transference towards the patient, including feelings directed at the patient based on the therapist's personal history, and his/her countertransference. The latter manifests itself when it is possible to identify which part of the patient's self is being placed inside the therapist's mind and provoking a reaction, idea or behaviour. In short, only the analyst's specific reactions towards the patient's particular qualities develop the specific concept of countertransference.

Grinberg (1956) provided a valuable contribution to the matter with his projective counter-identification concept, where the analyst responds by identifying with the patient's objects, and the phenomenon in which the analyst feels compelled to perform a role that has been projected into him/her. It is the violence of the patient's projective identification that, in addition to the analyst's unconscious conflicts, leads him/her to play such role. Grinberg's core idea is that in the projective counter-identification phenomenon the analyst does not participate with his/her conflicts and is taken over by the patient's projective process.

We then find that, over time, the countertransference concept gradually turned from an obstacle to treatment into an essential tool for psychotherapy practice. Besides, the disagreements between the totalistic and classic concepts decreased as time passed, and the totalistic view started earning greater support and agreement.

Gabbard (1995) highlights countertransference is an equally essential tool in analytic psychotherapy practice, despite some differences stemming from factors such as a lower frequency of sessions and the fact that patient and therapist are face to face. He believes that looking for, finding, and using countertransference are harder to do in psychotherapeutic practice than in the psychoanalytic practice.

Even today controversies exist on whether countertransference can encompass all of the therapist's reactions. However, there are no more questions regarding the importance of this concept as a helpful tool in the practice of psychoanalysis and psychotherapy, especially after the advances in theories about the analytic field.

The analytic field is a concept that represented an evolution in the studies about the patient's and the analyst's mind. As described by Baranger and Baranger, the analytic field

> is interplay of projective and introjective identifications, and their array of counter-identifications. . . . The situation is managed to avoid or limit the projective counter-identification phenomenon. The analytic situation comprises allowing the free play of projective identification in the patient, thereby giving him/her the exceptional chance to structure the couple fantasy according to his/her needs, with minimal resistance by his/her "partner" (Baranger & Baranger, 1969, p. 141)

The analytic field consists of the therapist–patient dyad and their transferential/countertransferential aspects pervade the entire situation of the analysis and describe how patient and analyst are always mutually influencing each other and interacting. The analytic field reveals a psychoanalysis that aims towards intersubjectivity. The therapist–patient dyad is no longer the sum of two people or two views of the world and treatment, but something new created in this union. In the case illustrated, we see how the analytic field can be set up differently when male-to-female gender dysphoria patients are seen by male therapists and when they are seen by female therapists.

The analytic field concept allows us to think that the problems that arise in the analytic relationship in a bi-directional manner are not due to the patient's or the therapist's responsibility, to the resistance by one or the other. They represent a specific pathology of an intersubjective structure resulting from cross-transferences and projective identifications and counter-identifications the dyad gradually expresses.

Enactments usually occur in this intersubjective structure. Enactment indicates aspects of psychic reality expressed in behaviours, gestures, or expressions that reveal unconscious obstructions or problems in one's verbal and symbolic expression skills. Characterised by acts, enactment is etymologically described by McLaughlin:

> The verb "act" is set between two modifiers. By itself, "act" . . . carries the meaning of "act", "do", "act one's will by force", "exert power", "perform as an actor to simulate or dissimulate" (play the role of); . . .

> The prefix "en" emphasises "act" as a noun, and conveys "putting into or upon, to wrap in, make like," adding a more intensive force; the suffix "ment" further intensifies the import and density of "act" as a noun (McLaughlin, 1991, p. 597)

Cassorla (2007) presents the idea of the therapeutic relationship as a space–time situation in which feelings, sensations, and thoughts between the members of the analytic dyad can be seen "enacted", as in the theatre. Scenes are put together and plots unveiled with significant expressions of what has been experienced/suffered to be worked on. Hence, he proposes using the expression "the analytic dyad in scene" to expand the understanding of the term enactment.

Countertransference in gender dysphoria

Gender dysphoria patients usually see doctors to get hormone therapy and surgery. They hardly ever seek psychological care. As a rule, the physician or assisting team is the one suggesting counselling for the patient, and the patient usually accepts it believing it to be a pre-surgery requirement. Chiland (2000) notes that, in her clinical experience with transsexuals, one of the great issues in these patients' analytic psychotherapy is their total focus on their body and sex reassignment surgery, and the consequent attempt to avoid any psychological involvement associated to their problems. Many patients fully believe their primary problem is their bodies, and the psychological problems attributed to it are secondary to that fact, instead of the other way around.

These patients generally find it very hard to accept a psychological approach to their conflicts, and hardly ever talk about their childhood or past events in their lives. Chiland (1988) believes it is very important to make it clear that psychotherapy/psychoanalysis is not meant to issue a certificate for the surgery but, instead, to help patients understand themselves and handle the difficulties inherent to their decision, whatever it may be.

If these patients have anything in common, it is that they do not talk about their childhood, and their "forgetfulness" has nothing to do with repressing or having amnesia about a childhood neurosis. It is organised forgetfulness. They tell a fabricated story to make sure they get what they want—gender reassignment surgery and hormone therapy—according to the "recipes" they see in the media or from other transsexuals. Hakeem (2012) also finds that it is not uncommon for patients initially to try to offer an "official version" of their stories, a copied and pasted version they prepared to fit what they believe professionals want to hear and so gain access to the physical treatment.

Gender dysphoria patients also tend to extinguish the past of their minds in which they lived as a member of the opposite sex, be it in their family context, at school, or in their own bodies. Chiland (2000) does not see that as a repression but, instead, as a split preceded by such desire wipe out the past.

Therapists treating transsexuals are in a very different position. They have their concepts of masculinity and femininity that immediately cause them reactions and constitute a serious countertransferential problem.

Lothstein (1977b) said that many gender dysphoria patients see psychological treatment as an obstacle to, or refusal of, surgery and internalise their therapists as persecutors. They might remain quiet during sessions, blocking and refusing to provide clinical material, or are highly invested in some superficial, unproductive narcissistic material. The therapeutic alliance is greatly compromised when the patient believes the therapist means to solve his/her problem in a non-surgical manner, which causes the patient's sense of urgency and hopelessness to increase.

Therapists cannot take it upon themselves to persuade the patients to have or not have surgery. Patients have their life goals that might or might not be achieved. Additionally, patients are extremely suspicious in these circumstances and "drop out" when they feel there is some opposition to their plans. At the same time, therapists cannot remain emotionally indifferent to the mutilation sought by the patients.

Therapists are very often seen as "judges" with respect to gender reassignment surgeries, which could lead to a belief that they play a double role as judge and persecutor while, at the same time, needing to know more about the patients' frailties. Therapists can also be seen as "transphobic" for offering psychotherapy instead of surgery/hormone therapy.

Lothstein (1977a) says that therapists choosing to treat gender dysphoria using conventional psychotherapy will find the patients' most significant understanding emerges from the analysis of countertransference. In group therapy, Lothstein (1979) found that these patients' emotional connection ranged between intense hostile dependency and the absolute absence of a relationship. Significant object relationships were non-existent. The sessions were superficial and shallow, and he was never able to take a deeper look at the issues. Close interpersonal contact was feared by the transsexual ego and led to fits of anger and flight. The patients' clothes, make-up, and appearance became substitutes for their lack of communication or inability to have emotional relationships with another person.

Lothstein (1977b) further divides the reactions according to the therapist's sex and the patient's gender. In this section, we illustrate a male therapist and a male-to-female patient. Male patients dressing as women (lipstick, bra, high-heeled shoes) might awaken intense feelings in the therapist. These feelings vary considerably and include: (1) cognitive dissonance regarding the sex and gender confusion; (2) envy of the opposite sex; (3) superego conflicts; (4) homosexual concerns; (5) defences against passivity and emotional surrender. In the early stage of their transition, these patients might convey a bizarre appearance while they experience intense narcissistic needs to be admired by the therapist. That reveals itself as a control strategy by the patient that could evoke a masochistic observance in the male therapist, and the latter might submit to the patient's demands due to both a cognitive confusion and a desire to be liked.

In the evaluation, evolution, and treatment of the male-to-female patient, the therapist's sexual preference (especially when it is for women) is highly important. The notions the male therapist has of a "real woman" will influence his clinical considerations and the patient's evaluation. The patient will naturally enjoy greater acceptance when he looks more like his gender identity.

The therapist's attitudes towards women and his views about femininity are decisively important in his evaluation of the patient's ability to play the role of a woman and express his femininity. For instance, a patient once heard the following words as he got to the emergency room at a general hospital, "How do you expect to be a woman? You are ugly and fat!!", meaning that fat and ugly looks are not compatible with femininity.

The therapist's anxieties about his own gender identity might remain on the surface as a strong negative countertransferential reaction, and the therapist's superego-related concerns might be projected into the patient.

Male-to-female patients are known to be provocative and seductive towards their therapists. Patient reports of scabrous sexual exploits with other men who were used, manipulated, and cheated can awaken fears, concerns, and a feeling the therapist might also be victimised by the patient, now seen as an impostor.

Lothstein (1977b) divides the transformation of the therapist's relationship with a gender dysphoria patient into five stages. These stages are: (1) voyeurism; (2) cognitive confusion; (3) denial and detachment *vs.* over-identification; (4) consolidation of the therapist's gender role; (5) working on the therapeutic process.

In the initial stage, when the patient is more exhibitionist (usually as a manifestation of behaviours he learnt from other patients or the media), the therapist needs to "fight" his diagnostic urge, his own values, and a premature tendency to accept/reject the patient and his needs. Therapists need to deal with ambivalent feelings of curiosity, excitement, and interest in the patient's presentation and appearance, which is usually bizarre. Therapists with superego conflicts and strong prohibitions related to looks might experience intense guilt leading to fantasies of punishment and retaliation.

In the second stage, the therapist might become confused as to the pronouns he uses to address the patient and finds himself in a state of disorganisation regarding the patient's problems. This confusion is often manifested by states of boredom, tiredness, or hostility directed towards the patient.

In the third stage, there is a polarisation between two therapeutic strategies, denial and the detachment against the over-identification. The first, in which the therapist attempts to take a non-critical, non-judgemental stance and accepts the patient's problems, might occasionally cause the emergence of anxiety, somatic symptoms, and micro-dissociative states, especially when the therapist is accepting anti-ethical behaviours and pathologies that go against his own values.

Therapists treating gender dysphoria might be subject to sadistic interventions. These sadistic fits might not be apparent at first, but can be noticed in a retrospective analysis. Therapists must be prepared to keep a non-judgemental stance that is welcoming of patients and their families. However, accepting the patient via a mechanism of over-identification with his conflicts could lead to sub-treatment and sub-diagnosis.

The fourth stage involves the reactivation of the therapist's own gender conflicts. Through the mechanism of empathic regression or empathic over-identification, a therapist exposed to the patient's identity conflicts realises that previously consolidated conflicts and resolved neurotic aspects of his sexuality might be reactivated as a conflict faced by the therapist himself. The reaction could be one of anger and hostility towards the patient.

The fifth stage is characterised by the establishment of the therapeutic alliance in which the therapist is more accepting of the patient in a more realistic manner, and manages to handle the conflicts that emerge in the treatment. Feeling more connected to the patient leads the therapist to behave more empathically towards the patient and be capable of helping the latter with his magical expectations and fantasies about the surgery.

Lothstein (1977b) concludes that it is productive to deal with the intense feelings aroused, considering that the therapists' natural reaction to such feelings is to grant the patients their wish to have the surgery and discontinue the psychotherapy, and that confronting countertransference with patients leads to lower dropout rates.

Clinical material and discussion

The clinical material described below comes from the psychotherapy treatment of a male patient seeking gender reassignment surgery to become a female, seen at the psychoanalytic psychotherapy outpatient clinic at the Psychiatry Service of Hospital de Clínicas de Porto Alegre (HCPA), connected to Universidade Federal do Rio Grande do Sul. This outpatient clinic at HCPA includes a clinic specialising in counselling gender identity disorder patients (PROTIG), which offers treatment for people to adapt to their desired gender. The first stage includes a hormone and behavioural approach. In cases where there are progress and recommendations, gender reassignment surgery is then offered. The accompaniment includes psychiatric and psychological assessments, and these patients are offered analytic psychotherapy. Similar to what is found in the literature, most patients see psychotherapy from a predominantly schizo-paranoid standpoint and fail to make the most of it as they believe that once their innermost beliefs and ambivalences become known, the recommendation for gender reassignment surgery will be denied. Supervising this case and other cases has particular characteristics because a network of projective and introjective identifications is established between the attending resident, the patient, and the supervisor that often reveals aspects of the analytic field and countertransference, as well as successive enactments.

In this gender dysphoria patient's psychotherapy, it was clear that he saw questions about this past as an investigation looking for clues to refute his "version" of being a woman in a man's body, and, therefore, he avoided talking about the subject. This attitude by the patient early on in the treatment left the therapist feeling self-conscious about once again looking into the subject of sexuality in childhood/adolescence. In retrospect, that might have been a way for the patient to control the sessions and avoid talking about things about which he was not sure.

In the course of the treatment, we also noticed how superficial and body-centred the sessions were, in addition to the low motivation to look deeper into important personal conflicts. That caused a strong sense of confusion that, combined with the therapist's lack of experience in the matter, made it seem as though the therapist was unable to understand what the patient wanted to communicate.

Additionally, there was a constant sense that the patient wanted to portray an image of femininity to society (and to the therapist) by adopting stereotypical behaviours to which the patient clung while overlooking his actual problems. That also made the therapist feel bored and often kept him in the role of a mere observer submitting to the patient's demands, owing to both a cognitive confusion and a desire to be liked, similar to what Lothstein had described.

In some sessions, the therapist felt clearly attacked, at times by the ironic tone the patient would take and at others by her threats to mutilate or hang herself in case her demands were not met. It seems clear she saw the clinic providing the sex-change surgery and the therapist as obstacles to her achieving her goal of having the surgery. Consequently, she deemed them trans-phobic and insensitive towards her situation. This paranoid stance often left the therapist paralysed, subdued by the patient's projections, and afraid to make interventions that might arouse her rage and allow the session to get out of control.

In other sessions, the therapist realised he was angry with the patient, in part because she denied reality and the fact that she had been born a man, but also because she put the therapist in the place of future partners (heterosexual men) being deceived by her assertions of being a woman born without a womb. Those assertions made her seem like an impostor.

Final considerations

The material described shows the countertransference difficulties faced when therapists are seen by patients as someone playing a double role. In this case, the patient fantasises the therapist is someone capable of either authorising a demand by the patient or not, instead of as an ally to help her understand her conflicts. In addition, it is clear this double role as judge and therapist is a source of these patients' hate of, and resistance towards, the therapist.

The clinical case and the literature cited show how useful the analysis of countertransference can be in these situations, and sometimes it is the only way to access the conflicts of such resistant patients whose capabilities for insight are compromised.

Lothstein (1977b) believes that acknowledging and interpreting the countertransference not only facilitates the therapeutic alliance, but also reveals core, essential issues for the patient (which are usually concealed from the therapist), and that a therapeutic alliance becomes impossible without the interpretation of countertransference.

Considering countertransference is essential in all analytic and psychotherapeutic efforts, it often becomes the decisive element in the treatment of patients with extremely serious difficulties, as is the case of gender dysphoria patients. That is why being mindful of one's own emotional reactions and using this monitoring to understand what the patient is trying to arouse in the therapist can represent the borderline between the possible failure or success in these treatments. Additionally, as it is present both in psychoanalysis and psychoanalytic psychotherapy, we need to keep on sharing clinical experiences and theories that allow us to advance more confidently into this new territory.

References

American Psychiatric Association (2013). *Diagnostic and Statistical Manual of Mental Disorders: DSM-5* (5th edn). Washington, DC: American Psychiatric Association.

Baranger, W., & Baranger, M. (1969). *Problemas del Campo Psicoanalitico*. Buenos Aires: Kargieman.

Cassorla, R. M. S. (2007). Del baluarte al enactment: el "no-sueño" en el teatro del análisis. *Revista Brasileira de Psicanálise, 41*: 51–68.

Chiland, C. (1988). Enfance et transsexualisme. *Psychiatrie de L'Enfant, 31*: 313–373.

Chiland, C. (2000). The psychoanalyst and the transsexual patient. *International Journal of Psychoanalysis, 81*: 21–35.

Eizirik, C. L., & Lewkowicz, S. (2014). Contratransferência. In: R. W. Aguiar, C. L. Eizirik, & S. S. Schestasky (Eds.), *Psicoterapia de Orientação Analítica* (pp. 300–309). Porto Alegre: Artmed.

Etchegoyen, R. H. (1987). *Fundamentos da Técnica Psicanalítica*. Porto Alegre: Artmed.

Fisk, N. (1973). The how, the what, the why of a disease. In: D. Laub & P. Gandy (Eds.), *Proceedings of the Second Interdisciplinary Symposium on Gender Dysphoria Syndrome* (pp. 7–14). Palo Alto, CA: Stanford University Press.

Freud, S. (1910d). The future prospects of psycho-analytic therapy. *S. E., 11*: 127–136. London: Hogarth.

Freud, S. (1912e). Recommendations to physicians practising psycho-analysis. *S. E., 12*: 111–120. London: Hogarth.

Gabbard, G. O. (1995). Countertransference: the emerging common ground. *International Journal of Psychoanalysis, 76*: 475–485.

Grinberg, L. (1956). Perturbaciones en la interpretación por la contraidentificación projectiva. *Revista de Psicoanálisis, 14*: 23–30.

Hakeem, A. (2012). Psychotherapy for gender identity disorders. *Advances in Psychiatric Treatment, 18*: 17–24.

Heimann, P. (1950). On coutertransference. *International Journal of Psycho-analysis, 31*: 81–84.

Hirschfeld, M. (1923). Die intersexuelle Konstitution. *Jarhbuch fuer sexuelle Zwischenstufen* [*the Yearbook for Sexual Intermediate Stages*], 23: 3–27.

Kernberg, O. P. (1965). Notes on countertransference. *Journal of the American Psychoanalytic Association, 13*: 38–56.

Lothstein, L. M. (1977a). Psychotherapy with patients with gender dysphoria syndromes. *Bulletin of the Menninger Clinic, 41*: 563–582.

Lothstein, L. M. (1977b). Countertransference reactions to gender dysphoric patients: implications for psychotherapy. *Psychotherapy: Theory, Research and Practice*, *14*: 21–31.

Lothstein, L. M. (1979). Psychodynamics and sociodynamics of gender-dysphoric states. *American Journal of Psychotherapy*, *33*: 214–238.

McLaughlin, J. T. (1991). Clinical and theoretical aspects of enactment. *Journal of the American Psychoanalytic Association*, *39*: 595–614.

Ruiz, P., Sadock, B. J., & Sadock, J. S. (2014). *Synopsis of Psychiatry* (11th edn). Philadelphia, PA: Wolters Kluwer.

Sandler, J., Holder, A., & Dare, C. (1970). Basic psychoanalytic concepts: counter transference. *British Journal of Psychiatry*, *117*: 83–88.

World Health Organization (WHO) (2010). International statistical classification of diseases and related health problems: ICD-10 (10th edn). Geneva: World Health Organization.

CHAPTER FOURTEEN

Neo-sexualities and the binary model debate[1]

Susana Muszkat

A young married man takes his baby daughter to the paediatrician for the first time. The receptionist greets him, and, as she fills out the patient's form, she asks, "Are you the father of this baby?" "Yes", he answers proudly, and she asks right away, "Name of the mother?" "She doesn't have a mother, she has two fathers", he states firmly. He had been bracing himself for this question since he and his husband embarked on the project of having a child. A sense of embarrassment follows—the receptionist's and that of other people present. The scene is unconventional, and, hence, disconcerting. The receptionist has no personal, symbolic, or emotional record of it because it is new to her. So she answers, "Oh, how nice!" in an attempt to restore balance to her frame of reference.

When he recounts this situation (unprecedented both for him and for the other people there) to me, who has been working with him for several years and has witnessed how he takes care of his daughter—his "primary maternal preoccupation" (Winnicott, 1958), his connection with, and attention to, the needs of this baby, his tales of everyday family feelings, anxieties, fears—I answer with a question that prevails on me as absolutely essential: "But do you actually think that your daughter doesn't have a mother?"

What do we mean when we say that someone does not have a mother? Our representation of a motherless child is that of a child who is missing the person who is indispensable for his mind, for his subjectivity to develop. The mother is the person who is responsible for providing the holding environment, for performing the reverie function. In other words, he or she must be capable of containing or incorporating the anxieties, violent drives, and frustration of the child and, in this way, provide the child with the necessary conditions to develop a thinking apparatus and to tolerate and transform sensations into meaning. Furthermore, the mother is the person responsible for taking care of the baby in the state of absolute dependence and basic helplessness that is inherent in the human condition—the person whose absence would lead to the baby's death, as Freud (1921c) claimed.

Yet, if my patient provides this baby with all of this, how can the assertion that the baby has no mother be justified? This development opened the door to new and interesting questions. My patient and I started talking about his experiences, for which there are no truths or consolidated models in our culture, and tried to find answers that made sense to him. This is new, uncharted territory that we are building, examining, and pondering in sessions over time.

Academic authors concerned with gender studies, as well as some psychoanalysts, have made interesting contributions to the topic of neo-sexualities. McDougall coined this term in 1986 to describe sexual practices observed in her consulting room that evinced the need to create specific, indispensable erotic scenarios that were unique and highly invested. The literature on this topic is speculative and inconclusive. Its main merit is that it brings to light and discusses the various possibilities of expression of humanness in terms of both the construction of identity and orientation in object choice.

I advance the notion of neo-sexualities in the current social context to designate the wide range of expressions of sexuality—the various forms of emotional connection that are not restricted to the binary system of heteronormativity. In this sense, I understand neo-sexualities as modes of expression of subjectivity that satisfy the subject-of-desire in those aspects that are authentic and unique to each person, in other words, that are not compelled to follow models that have been naturalised as healthy by hegemonic culture.

It is in this sense that Butler (2004) discusses the trans (transgender, transsexual) question, an issue that is complex and has generated controversy within as well as outside trans communities. Gender here should be understood as *gender identity*, a self-ascribed designation (as are reports on race and colour in census questionnaires) that transcends the notions of male and female. Gender identity operates in a context of political conflict that includes the entire (wide) spectrum of "trans" positionings as subjects' ways of existence. Butler explains that transgender becomes the term used broadly and loosely in everyday life by those who identify as men (if from female to male) or women (if from male to female), whether or not they have undergone sex reassignment surgery or hormonal treatment. What predominates is the singularity of sexualised bodies and desire.

These groups belong to a social stratum that suffers greater exclusion and discrimination than the gay and lesbian populations, and pathologisation is the main mark of their segregation from the broader normative system. Such difference might be due to the earlier development of gay and lesbian political movements, which granted these populations, if not full social approval, certainly the recognition and rights protection owed to them by virtue of their status as citizens.

To add to the matter, data obtained from a lengthy in-depth critical study of the literature on male same-sex parenthood published between 1979 and 2011 (Gato & Fontaine, 2014) show the complex meaning of standing outside the normative social trend. Prejudice faced by gay fathers stems from both external (social–cultural–family) and internal (intrapsychic) stereotypes. Some of the external stereotypes are the following: men are less connected to their children, and, therefore, less competent than lesbians, they have less talent for taking care of babies than women, and, even more, there is a risk of paedophilia, and lasting emotional relationships are unstable. In addition, LGBT groups are prejudiced against gay men who follow a model that has been traditionally viewed as heterosexual.

As to internal prejudice, the research discussed by Gato and Fontaine shows that gay fathers feel inadequate and suffer because they do not fit into the prevailing social pattern. They experience a conflict between an ego ideal supported by the social model, and their true needs and wishes. The authors refer to a study conducted by Berkowitz and Marsiglio (2007): "In this way, in entering a traditionally feminine domain, men who play a parental role without the presence of a woman violate traditional expectations regarding the male gender" (Gato & Fontaine, 2014, p. 314).

We certainly think of mothers as women; it has always been that way. We call a father who is affectionate a "fother",[2] or even "a father who is a mother". Is it time to revisit these appellations? Language has no way to designate arrangements that are new to us. Born from a lack, language must invent new names, for we are dealing precisely with a lack.

In the same way, psychoanalytic literature on neo-sexualities is still scarce. We find, however, mainly in link theory, the notion of an expanded psyche where the constitution of the subject unfolds in the complex interplay of the intrapsychic, the interpsychic, and the transsubjective, that is, what is transmitted through culture. The idea of an expanded psyche provides us with critical resources to ponder these new phenomena within the realm of psychoanalysis without having to relegate them to the field of social psychology or sociology. Even so, we are faced with questions derived from new problems, like the ones I pose here based on clinical vignettes.

It should be added that the above-mentioned review of the research on same-sex parenting concludes that while there are few studies on families formed by gay men, these families show that there is no reason for society to be concerned or alarmed (p. 319). This is also what Roudinesco (2003) asserts in *Família em desordem* [Family in Disorder].

Thinking outside the box

Several psychoanalytic thinkers alert us to the danger of feeling tempted to examine these new situations through the lens of well-established theories with which we identify and on which we base our psychoanalytic identity (McDougall, 1986; Mondzrak, 2008; Puget & Muszkat, 2009). By doing so, we risk compromising the essential aspects of psychoanalytic observation and listening, that is, openness to the new and the construction of meanings that are legitimate for each individual in the unique context of the experienced scene. It is thanks to such openness that we can give patients the freedom to experience and act in the world in tune with themselves.

Since McDougall's first conceptualisations, neo-sexualities have forced psychoanalysts to hone their theoretical tools in order to account for their clinical experience. McDougall already stated in 1986,

> By the same token, theoretical advances are the fruit of innumerable clinical experiences that have stimulated us to recognise theoretical impasses and to question our existing concepts. In addition, there is the ever-present risk that our theoretical beliefs unduly influence our technique so that our analysands may employ much of their analytical process in an attempt to confirm their analyst's theoretical expectations! (McDougall, 1986, p. 1)

Concerning the study of homosexualities, Ferreira Leite Neto (2014) claims in a recent article that psychoanalysis

> must be preserved and protected in its radical specificity. Studying the issues raised by homosexuality offers us a chance to ask questions. I believe that the instrumentalisation of psychoanalysis at the service of different forms of moralism is unacceptable and must be combated. (p. 88, translated for this edition)

As far as I am concerned, I would like to suggest that neo-sexualities, which include all transgenders as well as same-sex parenting, force analysts to think outside the box while firmly anchored in both the analytic method and in a conception of an expanded psyche.

Since I finished my Master's degree, I have felt the need to incorporate the cultural dimension into the psychic realm. At that time, I had coordinated male discussion groups on gender for ten years at an NGO that worked with families experiencing violence. I had learnt that, whether the perpetrator was male or female, violent practices could not be understood without taking social and cultural representations into account. By choosing the Social Psychology Department at the University of São Paulo, I attempted to bring together already acquired psychoanalytic tools, on the one hand, and the study of cultural issues and their paradigms and their influence on individual subjectivation, on the other.

Gender relations studies have created a space to conceive of an expanded psyche that is subjected and constituted by three agencies: the intrapsychic, the intersubjective, and the transsubjective, that is, culture. The patient whose story opens this essay has forced me to ponder and query what it means to be a father or a mother from a psychoanalytic perspective. This chapter offers more questions than answers.

Deconstructing models and producing broadened reconstructions

In the early 1960s and 1970s, the emergence of feminist movements, women's increased contribution to household income, and the appearance of the pill and the consequent dissociation between sexuality and reproduction revolutionised the model of the so-called "modern family". This model, which had governed male-female relations until then, gave way to what came to be called the "contemporary" or "postmodern" family (Roudinesco, 2003).

Gay and lesbian movements followed in the 1980s. In the context of the spread of AIDS and the consequent deepening of gender relations studies, these movements advocated for the deconstruction of traditional cultural values, which determined what was conventionally considered "natural" or "typical" for men and women (Muszkat, 2011). Gender studies have questioned the naturalness of some notions that are deeply ingrained in culture, such as heterosexuality and the status assigned to the feminine due to women's role in reproduction. In other words, they have challenged both the status and the role naturally assigned to men and women based on their biological make-up and their reproductive capacity (Muszkat, 2011).

There seems to be an agreement among psychoanalysts regarding the fact that subjects cannot develop without an other to subjectivise them. Yet, the naturalised belief that this other must be a female-gendered mother should be called into question. In her controversial book, *The Myth of Motherhood*, Badinter (1981) already casts doubt upon the well-propagated and instituted maternal instinct. This author wonders if such instinct is inherent in the female condition or is a socially and historically constructed myth. If the latter is the case, what is its purpose?

The patient in the example offered above is maternal, even if he is a man from a biological point of view. Desire *vs.* biology? Drive *vs.* instinct? Since he is biologically male, he has no eggs. Yet, neither does a woman whose age is incompatible with pregnancy, to whom her doctor suggests that she resort to *in vitro* fertilisation using her husband's sperm and a donor's egg. The baby's genetic code will be a combination of her husband's and the unknown donor's codes. The mother's genes will not be part of the baby. Genetics and new reproductive procedures belong in the realm of biology; the desires to have a child and form a family do not. From a biological viewpoint, the woman and the young man are in the same situation.

While Freud always strove to find a biological basis to support his constructions about the human psyche, his work also provides the clearest uncoupling of the biological and exogenous from the symbolical, the world of representations, which is manifested through phantasies, dreams, parapraxes, and symptoms. A body that is exclusively ruled by biology is not a human body; the human body is driven by desire and activated by drives.

Laplanche already questioned Freud's notion that the subject is initially centred upon himself, and challenged the idea of a phylogenetically determined nucleus of the unconscious (Hartke, 2014). Against the phylogenetic thesis, he asserted the essential presence of another in the constitution of human beings (Laplanche, 1997). According to Hartke (2014), "Laplanche . . . reestablishes the 'priority of the other' in psychoanalysis" (Hartke, 2014, p. 85, translated for this edition) and in the constitution of the subject. The matrix of subjects' unconscious, therefore, would be the unconscious messages transmitted by the adult carer and decoded, also unconsciously, by the child.

The input provided by this formulation, as I understand it, leads to the notion of an expanded psyche resulting from manifold determinations. This psyche is embedded in a web of transmission of both signified and non-signified elements that precede subjects and go beyond them. Coloured by their unique way of metabolising these elements intrapsychically, this web distinguishes each individual as unique and connected beings.

We are living once again in an age of "convulsed" paradigms. People's ways of relating, modes of family organisation, life projects, modes of production, work, human reproduction and affiliation, and ways of expressing their sexuality are being challenged. What is a mother? What does having a mother mean? What is a family? What does having a father mean? Or not having one and having two mothers instead?

Would the lack of a biologically male father undermine the logic of interdiction (the entry into culture), which presupposes the existence of a third? Can the notion of father implicit in the idea that it is the father who introduces the child into the world of law and belonging, a basic psychoanalytic concept be reduced to a biological definition? Or is this a concrete notion that is not consistent with that of representation? Is the paternal function assigned on the basis of biological features? (See also Minerbo, 2014.) Is the son of two mothers unable to enter the oedipal triangle? Are psychoanalytic theories in jeopardy as tools to understand human relationships? As psychoanalysts, we cannot deny human and world transformations in order to ensure the usefulness of our theories. Neither can we dispense with theories to avoid feeling obsolete.

Bleichmar (2014) suggests that we approach these issues based on a differentiation between the production of subjectivity and the constitution of the psyche. Let us take note of what she says:

> If we understand the *production of subjectivity* as historical, social, and political modes of instituting . . . forms of organisation of representational systems, the question is as follows: Which aspects of the psychoanalytic ideas and practices we have been carrying with us across a century of psychoanalysis have become dated in relation to current forms of production of subjectivity, and which are still valid in terms of the organisers of psychic functioning? (Bleichmar, 2014, p. 13)

In other words, we need to look at the persistence of theoretical models in relation to historical changes in modes of functioning.

The idea of sexuality and family was developed on the basis of a binary concept whereby differences were expressed through dichotomies, which are man/woman, homosexual/heterosexual, authorised/banned, and right/wrong. The binary condition favours one side of the pair over the other, and, hence, produces inclusions and exclusions. This perspective is not consistent with the intrinsic complexity of present-day families (Moscona, 2008). Like all analysts, I have analysands whose families vary in their composition. Some patients share the same parents with their siblings, others share only the father; there are stepmothers, stepfathers, fathers, mothers. . . .

A patient says to me, "I went on a trip with my family." "With your family?" I ask her. "Who was there?" "Me, my dad, his wife, and my little brother (their son)", she answers, "my dad's eldest son, and my half-brother on my mother's side". She immediately adds, "What a mess, right?"

In this comment, made by a young woman who is sophisticated and not at all conventional, I identify the traces of an ideal of family structure or makeup that places her on the other side of normative cultural values, that defines her as "outside the norm", a stranger, "outside the desirable". Normative values undermine her self-esteem, even though she reported having experienced immense pleasure in her outing with her "messy" family. Might her idealised expectations of a "non-messy", or normal, family constitute one of the obstacles that have been preventing this young woman from establishing creative, gratifying relationships?

To date, psychoanalysts have favoured the Oedipus complex as the major structuring factor in the development of individual subjectivity. It is this complex that instates the third in the dual baby–mother relationship, thereby marking the sexual difference between mother and father. The child is, thus, traversed by interdiction. This is the entry point into culture, the path towards the institution of a desiring subject (the subject of the lack) and towards symbol formation. If we take sexual differences into account, will this basic psychoanalytic concept collapse? I would like to refer once again to Bleichmar, who, while challenging the absolute nature of the Oedipus complex in terms of logics that are no longer exclusively guided by the phallic/castrated equation, highlights the ban on intergenerational *jouissance* contained in this concept, a ban that remains an indispensable constituting factor for the psyche (Bleichmar, 2014, p. 14).

Are differences determined exclusively by sex?

How can desire develop? Not desire of sex but of the other, of the other as different in his or her status of "alienness", a term coined by Berenstein and Puget (Berenstein, 2007), in his or her radical uniqueness. Moscona (2008) suggests that the paradigm of complexity leads to an expanded causality whereby the Oedipus complex is *just one* within a set of possible traces. In this way, subjectivity is constantly being developed on the basis of multiple norms. Kancyper (2004), in turn, opens new doors with his formulations about fraternal relations and generational differences, which give substance to these other traces.

In view of the multiplicity of potential family arrangements, how can we approach the various ways in which the psyche is structured and subjectivity is constituted? New arrangements imposed by subjects' desire favour temporary personal and love projects over traditional family projects. Modes of human reproduction also change;

sexuality and reproduction have been dissociated. Do children belong in a different register of desire? How should we understand this process?

"Whether we want it or not, other forms of relationship between the sexes emerge—new modes of partnership and affiliation, visible and legalized—in the world we inhabit", states Ferreira Leite Netto (2014, p. 82, translated for this edition). We find ourselves before an overwhelmingly disturbing new world. Interpersonal and link relationships have become more complex, and we are forced to challenge what had been conventionally thought of as "natural" and often understood as universal. Naturalisation imposes normative models that are incompatible with psychoanalytic thought.

Established, idealised hegemonic roles must be disrupted by incorporating new models in order to create new structuring factors. The expressions and manifestations of the sexual experience and the modes of affective connection deserving our attention are growing. Shall we have the courage to confront the threat posed by the need to dislocate and reconfigure our beliefs and values? Or must we sacrifice not only subjects in their original, unique practices, but also psychoanalysis?

Notes

1. Translated by Judith Filc.
2. *Pãe* is a neologism that combines the words for "dad" (*pai*) and "mum" (*mãe*), which is why I rendered it as "fother". (Translator's note)

References

Badinter, E. (1981). *The Myth of Motherhood: An Historical View of the Maternal Instinct*, R. de Garis (Trans.). London: Souvenir Press.
Berenstein, I. (2007). *Del ser al hacer. Curso sobre vincularidad* [From Being to Doing: A Course on Links]. Buenos Aires: Paidós.
Bleichmar, S. (2014). *Las teorías sexuales en psicoanálisis: qué permanece de ellas en la práctica actual* [Sexual Theories in Psychoanalysis: What Persists in Current Practice]. Buenos Aires: Paidós.
Butler, J. (2004). *Undoing Gender*. New York: Routledge.

Ferreira Leite Netto, O. (2014). Psicanalistas diante da questão homossexual: perplexidade? [Psychoanalysts faced with the homosexual question: Puzzlement?] *Revista Brasileira de Psicanálise, 48* (1): 81–92.

Freud, S. (1921c). *Group Psychology and the Analysis of the Ego. S. E., 18*: 67–145. London: Hogarth.

Gato, J., & Fontaine, A. M. (2014). Homoparentalidade no masculino: uma revisão da literatura [Same-sex male parenting: A review of the literature]. *Psicologia & Sociedade, 26*(2): 312–322. Available at www.scielo.br/pdf/psoc/v26n2/a08v26n2.pdf.

Hartke, R. (2014). Realidades e ficções na sexualidade e da sexualidade na psicanálise. Ficções fantasias e realidades [Realities and fictions in sexuality and of sexuality in psychoanalysis: Fictions, fantasies and realities]. *Revista Calibán, Realidades & Ficções, I*(*12*): 76–97.

Kancyper, L. (2004). *El complejo fraterno* [The Fraternal Complex]. Buenos Aires: Lumen.

Laplanche, J. (1997). The theory of seduction and the problem of the other. *International Journal of Psychoanalysis, 78*: 653–666.

McDougall, J. (1986). Identifications, neoneeds and neosexualities. *International Journal of Psychoanalysis, 67*: 19–31.

Minerbo, M. (2014). Assassinato e sobrevivência do pai [Murder and survival of the father]. Presented to the III Colóquio de Psicanálise com Crianças "Onde está o pai?" [Where is the Father?], Sao Paulo, October.

Mondzrak, V. (2008). Preconceito: razão e não razão [Preconception: reason and non-reason]. *Revista de Psicanálise da SPPA, 15*(1): 19–34.

Moscona, S. (2008). Lecturas actuales del Complejo de Edipo [Current readings of the Oedipus complex]. Presented to the II Conference on Psychoanalysis of Link Configurations, Argentina, May.

Muszkat, S. (2011). *Violência e Masculinidade* [Violence and Masculinity]. Sao Paulo: Casa do Psicólogo.

Puget, J., & Muszkat, S. (2009). Prejudice and social subjectivity. Paper presented at the 46th IPA Congress, 29 July–1 August, 2009, Chicago, USA.

Roudinesco, E. (2003). *A Família en Desordem* [Family in Disorder]. Rio de Janeiro: Zahar.

Winnicott, D. W. (1958). Primary maternal preoccupation. In: *Collected Papers: Through Paediatrics to Psychoanalysis* (pp. 300–305). London: Tavistock.

PART IV

TRIBUTE TO MARIAM ALIZADE

CHAPTER FIFTEEN

The liberation of parenthood in the twenty-first century

Mariam Alizade

The new forms of parenthood represent a potential revolution with respect to original paradigms of the psychoanalytic discipline. We need to rethink ideas accepted more than a century ago in order to renew theories and praxis and, thereby, encompass new forms of parentality in the twenty-first century. Introduction of the notion of function, both paternal and maternal, emphasised that it is not necessarily a biological mother or father who acts as such by virtue of the simple fact of being registered as such in filiation records. Another person may take this role and exercise this function.

Psychohistory, in turn, took up the task of revealing the dark side of parenthood. As Lloyd deMause writes (1974, p. 15, translated for this edition),

> The history of childhood is a nightmare from which we have begun to awaken quite recently. The farther we delve into the past, the lower the level of upbringing and the more exposed children are to violent death, abandonment, physical abuse, terror and sexual abuse.

The history of childhood in the Western world has developed in a more humanitarian direction since the eighteenth century, although filial violence and damage has not been eliminated. The compulsion to oppress and mistreat the weaker, abuse of power, and sadistic feelings of hate are frequently manifested in parents' relations with their children. The child is a symbolic character that influences all life, whether s/he materialises in parenthood, remains as a postponed project, is rejected, or is never realised.

The desired child is a depository of fantasies of transcendence, future protection when the parents will have grown old, symbolic survival, and reparation, among others. At the same time, the difficult child who defies narcissistic parental expectations provokes hostility and negative feelings in a sort of "tit for tat" in the link with feedback between reciprocally violent and destructive interactions.

The concept of generative identity proposed by Raphael-Leff (2003) defines the fragment of identity relating to the parental role. According to Raphael-Leff, this constellation of ideas concerning future parentality is found in children quite early in their development. Generative identity is the psychic construction of an individual as a potential parent.

The typical family, based on the father and mother as stable parents, was the ideal model of upbringing in the first hundred years of psychoanalysis. It seemed to be an immovable family model. Aberastury wrote (1984, p. 82), "All children need a father in order to detach themselves from the mother, and also need a father–mother couple to satisfy their bisexuality by projective identification". Salas (1984, p. 46) insisted on the importance of the existence of a real father in the parental couple for the exercise of this function. The heterosexual dyad was hegemonic and theories circulated on oedipal triangularity and narcissisation in the child's development.

In the twenty-first century, having a child is considered a human right, and the desire to form a family is strongly expressed in groups of neo-sexual, different, sexually unconventional persons. They are simply people who wish to build a nest of primary links beyond their gender identities or object choices. These expressions of wishes to generate a family organisation outside the social and cultural frame established centuries ago constitute a liberation movement. For these phenomena of novel parental inclusion, I propose the term: the liberation of parentality.

I have worked on the concept of the fourth complemental series (Alizade, 2004) in order to stimulate investigation of social, cultural, historical, and political factors in psychic organisation. Mandates and imperatives of the times in the external world are internalised in the mind through the superego, and they condition thinking and the creation of theories. The fourth series permeates the three complemental series described by Freud. Ideals, daydreams, fantasies, and desires, felt to be one's own, describe the dominant impregnation of culture, the subtle imposition of beliefs and of identification alienation. Apparent liberty of thought and action and the presumed authenticity of a wish are frequently subject to unconscious epochal conditioning.

In the same way that anatomy is destiny (Freud, 1924d, p. 178, quoting Napoleon), socio-cultural contexts form new destinies.

With the emergence of new parenthoods, requirements of an internal order have been established to evaluate a healthy adult project for bringing up a child. The fundamental elements for adequate parentality depend not only on external factors (marriage, heterosexuality, manifest desire for a child), but also on the mental health of the persons exercising the parental function, either together or as single parents.

Constitution as a heterosexual couple is no longer the fundamental element for bringing up a child. Capacity for love, sacrifice and responsibility occupy the foreground. Filiation takes a step backwards and the notion of natural maternity as being incarnated in all women has been questioned for several decades (Badinter, 1980).

In the light of these considerations, adoption acquires a positive, universal character. Universal adoption establishes that no parentality escapes the imperative of devotion and love towards the new being, whether biologically conceived or not. It implies that being adopted is synonymous with being loved and taken care of on the child's journey into adulthood.

The construction of a child (womb rental, purchase of sperm, etc.) due to technological inventions makes the panorama of parenthood even more complex. These gestations generate different fantasies and interactions. Father and mother acquire plurality: biological mother, sperm donor father, substitute mother, upbringing mother, symbolic father, etc. These multiple figures produced imaginary effects. For example, a father asks his adolescent daughter to lower the volume of her raucous music. The girl reluctantly obeys, exclaiming defiantly, "My donor wouldn't have asked me to lower the volume. I'm sure he would like to listen to this music." With these words, she introduced a hypothetical father of her own fabrication between her father and herself, an imaginary source of projections and desires.

There is no doubt that biological filiation weighs enormously on a child's upbringing and also that the desire for a child tends to be a narcissistic attractor of the highest order, in the sense of transcendence, generational continuity, imaginary and symbolic survival. We might even say that children brought up by a healthy and loving father and mother are privileged children and a model of excellent upbringing. However, the bare fact of being a father or mother implies neither health nor pathology. Each family organisation expresses its singularities. Wishing to be a father or mother may be—aside from an imperative of procreation and self-preservation of the species--a desire both healthy and pathological. The romantic vision of a nuclear family with children around contrasts with a multi-faceted parental reality. The desire for a child might become a tyrannical and narcissistic passion (Alkolombre, 2008) and the desire to not have a child could be a sign of maturity and responsibility.

I have explored the concept of family function with a research group in order to define which facts of life provide the child with access to the symbolic world and also to respond to new modalities of upbringing.

The family function denotes a network of subjectivities that support (or tear down) the psyche, in a branching arrangement of links that exceed the conventional nuclear family. In this network, biological filiations coexist with outside filiations. These are filiations with significant individuals who intervene in the child's map of identification and drive. They are people "outside the family" who produce psychic effects relevant to the child's mind and contribute to the structuring—or destructuring—of his or her psyche.

In this sense, as Viñar (2000, p. 322) states, "In order to make an individual, a group matrix is necessary. The 'we' precedes the 'I', the linguistic, affective, and identification thread conditioning individual behaviour and modelling it in each situation."

The word "family" expands to encompass persons, institutions, and groups. All the complexity of the adult world intervenes in the mental organisation of new generations. It is no longer limited to father and mother as the indispensable binomial in a child's gestation and upbringing.

The range of parenthoods has become more complex, with multiple divorces and children of different couples who form a new type of sibling relationship, halfway filiations (half-siblings), multiple stepfathers or stepmothers, and group territories that psychoanalysis is now investigating. Studies on links (Berenstein, 1991; Pichón Rivière, 1956–1957; Puget & Berenstein, 2001, among others) have contributed to develop novel concepts of interactive dynamics.

In the interest of protecting childhood and preventing disorders, society questions whether it should limit certain types of adoption. It asks for a guarantee of healthy upbringing for all new ways to exercise the care of a child.

Same-sex parenthoods are now in debate (Rotenberg & Agrest, 2007). On this point, I quote a fragment written a few years ago (Alizade, 2007):

> The exercise of homoparentality is eminently heterogeneous. It is impossible to homogenise either clinical situations or psychic consequences. Homoparental reproduction always requires the participation of a third party (a lender of the uterus, sperm donor, adoptant, etc.) in the reproductive encounter. Reproductive combinations now established were unimaginable when technology had not yet modified the ways to conceive a child. (p. 81, translated for this edition)

A kind of reproductive transsexuality occurs with an unconscious posture—or perhaps imposture—in an attempt to incarnate what will never be: the man a biological mother, the woman a biological father: an encounter analogous to the transsexual position that aspires to the impossible destiny of removing one sex from the body and placing the opposite sex into it. This point requires meticulous empirical investigations for clarification and consequent theorisation.

Heinemann (2006) has worked with clinical cases of children of homoparental couples. She postulates the existence of a universal mythical representation independent of the reality of the sex of each genitor. This author proposes the existence of a dividing line between adult sexuality and the child's psychosexual development that keeps childhood development independent of the genitors' gender.

According to McDougall (1995), since sexuality is polymorphous in all its manifestations, it cannot be considered perverse when it does not damage the other and is consented to by the participants in the sexual situation. In this perspective, a given neo-sexual person has the right to recognition and legal permission to adopt children, given that neo-sexualities are also heterogeneous and include people capable of taking care of and supporting an infant on the road of life towards adulthood.

In any case, any unlimited right to parentality concerns, frightens, and even provokes scandal, when potential genitors are considered strange or different.

The liberation of parentality represents a new liberation, just as women's liberation did in the nineteenth century; as such, it will have its advantages and disadvantages and will produce conflicts and controversies. It is a challenge for psychoanalysis. It deserves profound and unprejudiced, rigorous and interdisciplinary studies in relation to its psychic consequences for children and for the structure of society.

References

Aberastury, A. (1984). La paternidad. In: A. Aberastury & E. Salas (Eds.), *La Paternidad* (pp. 83–107). Buenos Aires: Kargieman.

Alizade, A. M. (2004). La cuarta serie complementaria. Unpublished.

Alizade, A. M. (2007). Pensando la homoparentalidad. In: E. Rotenberg & B. Agrest (Eds.), *Homoparentalidades. Nuevas Familias* (pp. 77–83). Buenos Aires: Lugar Editorial.

Alkolombre, P. (2008). *Deseo de Hijo, Pasión de Hijo*. Buenos Aires: Letra Viva.

Badinter, E. (1980). *L'Amour en Plus*. Paris: Flammarion.

Berenstein, I. (1991). Reconsideración del concepto de vínculo. *Revista de Psicoanálisis*, APdeBa, *XIII*(2): 219–235.

DeMause, L. (1974). La evolución de la infancia. In: *Historia de la Infancia* (pp. 15–92). Madrid: Alianza Editorial.

Heineman, T. (2006). Reconstructing Oedipus? Considerations of the psychosexual development of boys of lesbian parents. In: A. M. Alizade (Ed.), *Motherhood in the Twenty-first Century* (pp. 85–96). London: Karnac.

Freud, S. (1924d). The dissolution of the Oedipus complex. *S. E., 19*: 173–182. London: Hogarth.

McDougall, J. (1995). *The Many Faces of Eros: A Psychoanalytic Exploration of Human Sexuality*. New York: W. W. Norton.

Pichon Rivière, E. (1956–1957). *Teoría del vínculo, selección temática de transcripciones de sus clases*, F. Taragano (Ed.). Buenos Aires: Nueva Visión, 1985.

Puget, J., & Berenstein, I. (2001). *Psicoanálisis de la Pareja Matrimonial*. Barcelona: Paidós.

Raphael-Leff, J. (2003). La identidad generative. Conference on assisted reproduction given in APdeBA, Buenos Aires.

Rotenberg, E., & Agrest, B. (2007). *Homoparentalidades. Nuevas Familias*. Buenos Aires: Lugar Editorial.

Salas, E. (1984). El concepto de paternidad en algunos autores postfreudianos. In: A. Aberastury & E. Salas (Eds.), *La Paternidad* (pp. 29–47). Buenos Aires: Kargieman.

Viñar, M. (2000). Los niños fuera de la ley. La violencia de la exclusión, *Revista de Psicoanálisis*, Special International Issue, *7*: 317–329.

CHAPTER SIXTEEN

Alcira Mariam Alizade

Graciela Cardó Soria

With sorrow and surprise, we learnt that, on 6 March 2013, Mariam Alizade went ahead of us on the journey. What follows is a tribute, intended as a work of mourning. Mariam participated in several congresses and other activities of the SPP. She was, and still is, a benchmark for many of us. The legacy that she left behind: her books, COWAP, and all the traces of her life, to some extent fill the vacuum left by her early passing. This chapter is a biographical sketch of her life and some of her major theoretical contributions. We will cover three central themes that run through her work: femininity (*Feminine Sensuality*), death (*Clínica con la Muerte*) and positivisation (*Psychoanalysis and Positivity*). The first one introduces fundamental concepts such as "women-only" space, "intrapsychic maternalisation", and "non-maternal psychic space". The second one enables us to think about our death, introduces different concepts of dying and living, and develops the concept of "tertiary narcissism". The third one turns the positive dimension into a concept and introduces what Alizade termed the "psychic, that's it".

"Yo pido luz cada día, porque cada día es día magnífico para vivir y morir" [Every day I ask for the light because every day is a great day to live and die] (Alizade, 2012[1995]).

Who was Mariam?

Alcira Mariam Alizade, a physician and a psychoanalyst, was a member of the Argentine Psychoanalytic Association. In 1999, she was appointed the Latin American co-chair of the Committee on Women and Psychoanalysis of the International Psychoanalytical Association (COWAP) by the President of the IPA, Dr Otto Kernberg, and was then overall chair of COWAP from 2001 to 2005. She was scientific secretary of FEPAL from 2006 to 2008. Mariam Alizade, a woman proud to belong to the human species, passed away on 6 March, 2013.

According to her own words, she was born in Buenos Aires in July 1943 and grew up in "a very big house with a beautiful garden" in Belgrano, a traditional neighbourhood of Buenos Aires. Her arrival in this world happened earlier than expected, and she was delivered at home by an uncle who was a physician. Her father was Persian and her mother Argentinean of Spanish and English descent.

Her great-great-grandfather, Marcos Sastre, was a renowned educator and writer, founder of the first literary workshop in 1837. Her grandfather, Ali, owned a rug factory, first in Tabriz and then in Teheran, and it was he who taught her to know and love rugs.

She used to recall that, as a little girl, she would frequently visit her father's printing shop and play among letters and paper from different countries. One might think, based on all this information, that the ground was being laid for the future psychoanalyst and author: a big house that sheltered and nurtured her; many experiences that she started to treasure; letters and papers that would later become part of her life: poetry and writing. The colours and textures of her grandfather's hand loomed rugs, her diverse ancestors, her multi-culturalism and the many languages she would master provided her with the ability to understand and translate different languages from different people, in other words, to understand the nature of the unconscious. I would dare to say that her inner world was full of plenty of aesthetic experiences that would give her the characteristic delicacy and sensitivity that allowed her to perceive the nuances of the human soul and to understand the thousands of wefts the psyche is made up of.

Mariam Alizade was the middle child in a family of five children. She was well educated; she learnt German in primary school and French in high school. She also learnt English and took piano lessons. Her sensitivity was permanently being nurtured. It is easier, thus, to understand her three vocations: the writer, the teacher, and the physician; psychoanalysis allowed her to combine them.

She graduated at age twenty-four from medical school at Universidad Nacional de Buenos Aires. After a brief clinical period, she started analysis. Driven by a strong interest in deeply understanding the mysteries of the mind, she first entered training as a psychiatry resident and later served as an attending physician in the Psychopathology Service of Hospital Municipal Ramos Mejia for a short period. Just two years ago, she remembered attending patients in a hallway stuffed with small tables arranged one after the other, and being supervised in that hallway by Enrique Pichón Rivière, Justiniano Achával, and Nicholas Spiro, among other prominent psychiatrists and psychoanalysts. In her words, those were years of exciting scientific exchange and learning.

After seven years of practice as a psychiatrist, she earned her diploma and was accepted in the Argentine Psychoanalytic Association, from where she graduated a few years later. From then on and until her death, she continued giving seminars focused primarily on Freud's work.

She was supervised by Joyce McDougall, with whom she also had a personal relationship, and learnt a considerable amount, especially from the diligence with which she listened to the clinical material and the way in which she formulated relevant and intelligent questions, promoting reflection from various theoretical and clinical standpoints. Another mentor who inspired her work was Didier Anzieu, with whom she had a strong bond. In her words, "He was a privileged witness during the writing of the book (*Feminine Sensuality*) and we discussed various viewpoints. I visited him in his office in Paris about four times, and during our meetings we used to share ideas. I remember some exchanges we had about the end of the Oedipus complex in women and the concept of the stone core . . . He would say, 'I had never thought of that, how interesting!' or 'I had a patient who used to bring a small pebble to each session'. And then he would open a drawer and show me a number of jealously guarded stones."

Her first book, *Feminine Sensuality*, was published in 1992 (1999 in English) and translated into English and Italian. In her writings, she defined her three major areas of exploration, psychosexuality, death, and contemporary clinical work. In 1995, her second book, *Clínica con la Muerte* [Clinic with Death] was published. It sold out and is waiting for a second edition. Other publications were: *Tiempo de Mujeres* (Women's Time), *la Mujer Sola* (the Single Woman), *Psychoanalysis and Positivity* (translated into English), *Adiós a la Sangre* (Farewell to Blood), and *La Pareja Rota* (The Broken Couple). She also compiled many books in Spanish and English throughout her service on the Committee on Women and Psychoanalysis, from 1998 to 2005. Some titles are: *Motherhood in the Twenty-first Century; The Embodied Female; Studies on Femininity; Masculine Scenarios, Ser y Hacer de las Mujeres* [Women's Being and Doing]; *Psiconálisis y Género* [Psychoanalysis and Gender], *Escenarios Femeninos* [Feminine Scenarios]; *Masculino–Femenino* [Masculine–Feminine].

In her later works, she wrote about impermanence, happiness, and wellbeing, verbal incest, castration and finitude, parenthood liberation, living in the twenty-first century, homoparenting, the role of conscience in the analytic praxis, and the concept of intimacy in psychoanalysis.

Knowing Alizade in person also meant being familiar with her work. With simplicity, humility, and refinement, she embodied many of the concepts developed in her work: femininity, tertiary narcissism, the "women-only" space, and positivity. In the Intergenerational Dialogues between Men and Women, which Alizade promoted in Buenos Aires in 1999, there is an environment of freedom that fosters the generation and exchange of ideas that reflect cultural changes and their psychological impact, which was the central feature of her philosophy. Thus, I believe that not only did she theorise about and elaborate notions that help us understand the human psyche, but she also lived and transmitted those notions in her lectures, supervisions, and, principally, in her daily life.

Her contribution

In 2011, I had the chance to ask her what was her most cherished work, to which she replied: "All of them"; "Then tell me which one is the most representative one", I insisted, reformulating my question. After giving it a careful thought, she finally answered that it was "The end of the Oedipus complex in women" (In: *Feminine Sensuality*, 1999). Even though her contributions to psychoanalysis are broad, I will highlight three theoretical and clinical standpoints in this tribute:

women, death, and positivity, and unpack what these three concepts had in common for Alizade. To this end, I will briefly go over three books that I consider essential in her work: *Female Sensuality* (1999), *Clínica con la Muerte* (1995), and *Psychoanalysis and Positivity. Theoretical and Technical Implications* (2009).

On women

The subject of her book, *Feminine Sensuality* (1999), is clear from the title itself. Feminine sensuality differs from feminine sexuality. Sensuality is described as the sensory matrices that will be subsequently reframed. They are experiences that occur before the appearance of verbal expression and are, thus, a prevailing narrative of corporeal experiences. This concept reminds us of Klein's "memories in feelings" (1988), which become the basis of each woman's relational codes, basic and constitutive moments of the subject and his/her psyche, linked to the body in which we are and live. Then she describes Anzieu's contributions (1987), such as the different ways of thinking about, and understanding, the body: the body of affection, the erotic body, the body defined by language, the ethical body, the social body. These dimensions of the body take us back to Foucault's ideas (1984) about the discourses that permeate bodies, creating truthful evidence that limit the development of the ego.

In this body, which is the place where pleasure and displeasure occur, the sensual–affective weft resulting from multiple exchanges is consolidated; we could say that we are also referring to Kristeva's semiotic *chora* (1993).

The woman's body is the "preferred shape" (Alizade, 1999), since it is the primary body on which the first fundamental experiences are reflected; the initial desiring exchange is feminine and takes place in this "homosensual" field—we are referring to the primary relationship between two women that leads to the first structuring specularity. According to Lacan (1983), the concepts of primary narcissism, body and image, are intertwined. The concept of feminine sensuality opens the way for other theoretical developments. One of them is that of "giving oneself a body" (Alizade, 1999), which is a vital function that allows the development of the physical and psychic self.

Psychic and social, sensorial, aesthetic, erogenous, affectional, and ethical functions defined by language take place. The encounter between psyche and culture and between one person and another re-emerge. The author refers to maternity and to the primary relationship with another founding supporter of the psyche through love and protection.

The primary relationship with the mother, the mythic time of that "love bond" that implies the "body against body" contact, places the mother, or the one who is positioned in the place of the primary object, in a privileged place where the girl (Levinton, 2000) finds support for the imaginary belief in maternal omnipotence as a possible source of satisfaction for all her needs and, principally, for the containment of her anxieties. This first body against body contact opens, according to Alizade (1999), a first experience of the dimension of the "women-only" space between the mother and the girl. This dimension allows the formation of identifications via the encounter with the images of other women, so as to be able to "be" without any rivalries. The "body against body" concept takes us directly to Irigaray (1984), whose book, *El cuerpo a cuerpo con la madre* [The Body Against Body Bond with the Mother], discusses the importance that these early links with a being of the same gender have for women.

These particularities related to the development of the girl will make her an attachment being, as noted by Gilligan (1994), Chodorow (1984) and Levinton (2000). Alizade explains this, claiming that there is a

> seemingly inherent attachment to her feminine self due to the long period of pre-oedipal fusion with her mother, to the role played by the potential maternity understood as two bodies in one, and to the socio-cultural commands that have promoted her confinement to a private and dependent life through the ages. (2005, p. 167, translated for this edition)

From another standpoint, the achievement of the "women-only" space, which is the space where the first structuring specularity of initial feminine exchanges takes place, would relate to the concept of female genealogy developed by Irigaray (1984). This "women-only" concept is in line with the idea of the possibility of repair and recovery of the feminine genealogy, which necessarily involves the decline of the great primitive mother, the mourning of the omnipotent mother, who, as Chasseguet-Smirgel (1964) argues, is the result of a deep desire to detach herself from something divine. The girl, in the words of Chasseguet-Smirgel, has to develop a value of her own.

In *Ser dos* [To Be Two], Irigaray (1997) reminds us that continuing to be two means giving up childhood, in which one's omnipotence has prime importance; it means wanting to be an adult by relinquishing the needs of infancy. In the words of Alizade (1999), it means the girl accepting the mysteries of life and death, the mystery of creation, in a space that is different from her mother's.

We are entering a period of the decline of the Oedipus complex in women, the idea developed by Alizade in her book. Appealing to other myths such as Electra, or Demeter and Persephone, she depicts the positivisation of *no* in woman: she will have a vagina, a non-phallic order, the ability to be alone will appear, she will live in her own psychic space, and the so-called "intrapsychic mothering" will take place. The decline of the Oedipus complex in women will be a movement of affirmation.

Another important concept is that of the "stone core" (Alizade, 1999), which is a harsh, sexless inner space with a centre of gravity that supports the psyche. The author notes that imagination leads us to support the idea of a skeleton, or a frame, that gives uniqueness to the self. Alizade considers that before being male or female, one is a human being. She introduces the concept of human identity as that which precedes gender and that is present throughout life as a universal concept of existence (Alizade, 2005).

The stone core echoes the good object described by Klein, which constitutes the core of the ego and supports the mind throughout life's transit. By gradually being set in the mind, the core of the Kleinian good object/stone leads to profound transformations.

Another important contribution of Alizade's (2006) is the proposal of a "non-maternal psychic space" for women. She asks, "Can women's psyche be thought of outside the realm of motherhood?" (p. 52, translated for this edition). This implies a necessary dissociation between femininity and motherhood. The concept is linked to the stone core that rises above the corporeal body to where the transcendent and the sublime dwell.

On death

Saying that *Clínica con la muerte* [Clinical work with the dying] (1995) is a beautiful book might sound contradictory, but, as with life, Alizade presents interesting approaches to death, about which little has been theorised in psychoanalysis. Once again, clinical work opens up a door to theoretical work. Alizade emphasised that, due to our clinical work with living beings, we perceive the presence of death through the "mark of the mortal being that is always executed on its own flesh" (p. 37). Thus, the body imposes its "ever-living mortal presence" (p. 15).

The idea that "one will die" (1995, p. 33), opens the way to Alizade's thoughts about narcissism, the beginning of life, and its inexorable end. Dying is always reserved to the other, the stranger. The fact that one will die does not relate to oneself, or, at best, it will be deferred in time. It is always *someone else's death* that is the one that reminds one of oneself. The ego recreates its immortality from its unconscious roots.

Being able to think about death, we meet both extremes: those with the highest courage, who face the perishable nature of human existence, and those who are afraid of both death and life.

Bridges will be built from narcissism to reach the various ways of dying, which are masterfully described by the author. Imagine the poetic hand, a death protected inside a shell, a death giving away its skin, sharing silence that turns into wrapping, erotic deaths, thanatic deaths. A technical proposition arises: the "silent cure" (1995), which, for Alizade, is a complement to the Freudian "talking cure". She proposes it as a useful tool, taking into account the semiotics of silence that comprise various empathetic, closed, open, and painful meanings.

The silent cure is the pause of emerging sounds and words; it is the temporary or permanent quietness of the bustle of life; it is the mental space that occurs between the interruptions of words and phonemes. It corresponds to what Kristeva (1993) referred to as "the semiotic". It marks what the word has silenced or what has not even started to be registered in speech; it expresses in encrypted language what is barely decipherable. Referring to Wittgenstein, Alizade (1995) reminds us that "whereof one cannot speak, thereof one must be silent"; wise words, since death puts us on the threshold of silence.

It is in this context that a transcendental concept appears, we refer to "tertiary narcissism" (1995), which would account for the ways in which the human being is confronted with castration and finitude. It is the possibility of taking the social dimension into account, but the question promptly arises: will the cutting of primary, oceanic narcissism that allows the advent of the self be experienced primarily with sadness and pain, as described by Andreas Salome (1982), or, on the contrary, with the feelings of joy described by Lacan (1983) upon the recognition of the unified image? Probably both coexist, but the quality of the traces imprinted in "his/her majesty the baby" (Alizade, 1995), will determine the future development of the tertiary narcissism. It is about the relationship with the other, a stranger, an alien, a "faraway object" (Levinas, 2000). It recalls the notion of the purified pleasure-ego, discussed by Freud in his work "Negation" (1925h). It has to do with reversing these primary allocations towards the other. Tertiary narcissism would be the result of a structural transformation movement of the psyche, with clinical and social implications for the degree of control over the death drive and destructiveness. It has to do with passing from experiencing the other as the carrier of evil and strangeness to experiencing the sameness of the other as a close neighbour, who challenges us without being present. It reminds us of what that other ethicist, the philosopher, Emmanuel Levinas, spoke about (2000).

This tertiary narcissism will guarantee the future in which we will not live, just as in the story of the date sower, in which a neighbour asks him why he sows dates, considering they take so long to bear fruit that he would not live long enough to eat them. "Precisely", the man replies. Pleasure does not lie in sacrifice, which would be closer to moral masochism, but in the transformative possibilities of the life drive. It resembles the primary narcissism as it integrates into the world and goes beyond the subject; it is not great, it is not omnipotent; rather, it is finite, it knows about its own death, it goes beyond itself in a movement of transcendence.

From clinical work, Alizade reassesses the fact that we work with life, with Eros and Thanatos; we work with real losses that originate mourning and with imaginary losses that originate melancholy, but we also work with pre-death, with the death of our loved ones who are in a "departing status" (Alizade, 1995), with physical pain and psychic death. Thus, the drastic and radical death is unveiled in all its moments and levels; death that, according to Freud, does not exist in the unconscious turns then into a complex thing that comprises all the circumstances of the one dying when approaching the final moment: the environment that supports and sustains him/her or not, his/her pathology or health condition that allows him/her to be cocooned by others, his/her fantasies, his/her spirituality.

On contemporary psychoanalytic technique

In her book, *Psychoanalysis and Positivity: Theoretical and Technical Implications* (2009), Mariam Alizade makes contributions to technique, thereby promoting intense reflections and questions. She introduces the term "positivity" in psychoanalysis, giving it the category of concept. First, she notes that seriousness and suffering were, from the origins of psychoanalysis, categorised as important. On the other hand, joy and triviality were seen as insignificant psychic aspects. Disrupted associations, intolerable representations, unpleasant and repressed affects, pathology—all of them built the path that led Freud to his great discovery of the operation of the unconscious. None the less, dreams, jokes, slips of the tongue, and parapraxes were also considered by the founder of psychoanalysis.

That is how Alizade begins her proposition of considering positivity in psychoanalytic praxis. Poetically, she leads us to think about psychoanalytic treatment as the conquest of life-drive territories, as the appearance of the de-traumatising thought. She relies on the ability of the psychic apparatus to minimise conflict and bases her theory on Freud's (1950[1895]) *Project for a Scientific Psychology*, by describing the neuronal movements of facilitation, ramification, associative reflection, and infiltration.

Alizade explains the processes that occur in a session during the psychoanalytic treatment. She emphasises the role played by the persistent strength of an experience that can be modified through repetition, which explains the importance, in some cases, of session frequency. She develops the idea of reversing the sign of repetition (repetition of traumatic experiences and potential to reverse the sign of repetition and introduce repetitions of pleasant experiences). The notion of inner framing and the exploration of joy-related affects are discussed in other chapters of the book.

For Alizade, cure must involve the detoxification of the psyche from displeasure. It does not mean denying what is intolerable, but weaving it finely together with tolerable representations that will offer the possibility of putting a brake on re-traumatisation.

She alleges the presence of some analytical iatrogenesis when repetitive insistence on painful memories does not lead to elaboration and overcoming, and, instead, installs re-traumatising movements. Many patients end up believing that cure happens only through pain.

It is then that her proposition of the psychic "that's it" emerges (2009), which involves stopping negative rumination that involve will and consciousness work.

Our job "takes place in the dark night of the tragic hell as well as in the realm of desiring freedom and mental harmony" (Alizade, 2009, p. 78). She warns us that the stiffening of the frame is often in the service of an ideal technique that might oppose the patient's cure.

Quinodoz (1993) wrote *The Taming of Solitude*; Alizade, in turn, raises the idea of taming trauma, which involves symbolising tragedy so that the story receives representations and affections that will rectify and reorganise the psyche. Our expertise and our unconscious are put to work in an active and transforming intersubjective field.

This book invites us to evaluate our ethics and responsibility, as well as our empathy and limits.

Final comments

Mariam Alizade's contributions are not only scientific and experiential, but also institutional. As the first co-chair for Latin America of COWAP, she embodied the philosophy of this work group: simplicity, dialogue, the intergenerational issue and generativity. Psychoanalysis allows one to think about new families, new sexualities and the complexities of new parenthoods.

We are coming full circle. Hand in hand, Alizade has taken many of us down the road of human beingness, from birth and helplessness to death. During the tour, she paused to enquire about women, sensuality, psychosexuality, gender, family, neo-sexualities, menopause, and divorce. In beautiful and simple prose, she went from metapsychology to clinical work, and from there to technique, the positive and poetry as allies. With the originality of her ideas, she keeps us holding to the hope of developing a tertiary narcissism, elaborating the meaning of life in the continuum of history, and processing its loss and our own finitude.

Questioning the place of the tragic fate of human beings in order to arrive on the shores of happiness is still a no-go zone for a given sector of psychoanalysts. We must admit that, in many cases, people want to be happy; the life drive reigns over death. Without denying the necessary journey through Hades of "The Hero with a Thousand

Faces" (Campbell, 2004), Alizade dared—and many are grateful to her for that—to propose a "psychic that's it" by claiming that there is health, there are people who, in the words of Klein (1988), have a good object and, therefore, are balanced and have a capacity for sound judgement, and who are able to find satisfaction, peace, and sanity. They have internal resources and elasticity, as well as spiritual peace after experiencing great moral pain; they are full of gratitude for past pleasures and have the ability to enjoy what the present gives them. Serenity in life, as well as unembittered resignation, allows them to enjoy simplicity, something that is so often neglected. For Klein (1988), and Alizade (2006), the origin of all this is in childhood: it derives from the enjoyment of the breast without much envy of the mother, according to Klein, and the concurrence of bodies and sensory engrams in the body of affection, in the cocoon that allows survival. This origin is, nevertheless, complex when life circumstances and events are considered.

Even though there is a large proportion of female genealogies that are disrupted by body against body conflicts and hostilities, it is always good to refer to Alizade's lessons about positivity in psychoanalysis and to apply them to gender theory. Let us always keep in mind that there is mental health, that mothers with good milk do exist, as do fertile land and fallow land for the growth of the self and others.

Within the spectrum of her work, we find these significant themes: the mother, the body, and death. Men and women relate primarily to the mother. In his paper, "The theme of the three caskets", Freud (1913f) had already noted the importance of woman to men; she was so valued, feared, and envied that men divided her into three aspects.

Life is full of exchanges with the other that will generate and modify the psyche, facts of life that will mark bodies and souls. Alizade taught us that the challenge is to learn and, what is more, to transmit the art of living; so, in honouring her, I believe that we must remember we are part of the perishable. I conclude by recalling her saying, as we watched the Pacific Ocean, "And to think that we will pass away, that our life is nothing compared to the age of the sea . . . soon we will not be here and the little girl running over there will be old . . . we must enjoy life."

References

Alizade, A. M. (1995). *Clínica con la Muerte*. Buenos Aires: Amorrortu [reprinted Buenos Aires: Ed. Biebel, 2012].

Alizade, A. M. (1999). *Feminine Sensuality*. London: Karnac.

Alizade, A. M. (2005). *Adiós a la sangre. Reflexiones psicoanalíticas sobre la Menopausia*. Buenos Aires: Lumen.

Alizade, A. M. (2006). Motherhood in the Twenty-First Century. London: Karnac.

Alizade, A. M. (2009). *Psychoanalysis and Positivity: Theoretical and Technical Implications*. London: Karnac.

Andreas Salomé, L. (1982). *El narcisismo como doble dirección*. Barcelona: Tusquets Ed.

Anzieu, D. (1987). *El yo piel*. Madrid: Cátedra.

Campbell, J. (2004). *The Hero with a Thousand Faces*. Princeton & Oxford: Princeton University Press.

Chasseguet-Smirgel, J. (1964). *La sexualidad femenina*. Madrid: Biblioteca Nueva.

Chodorow, N. (1984). *El ejercicio de la maternidad*. Barcelona: Gedisa.

Foucault, M. (1984). *Historia de la sexualidad 2: El uso de los placeres*. México: Siglo XXI.

Freud, S. (1913f). The theme of the three caskets. *S. E., 12*: 289–302. London: Hogarth.

Freud, S. (1925h). Negation. *S. E., 19*: 235–241. London: Hogarth.

Freud, S. (1950[1895]). *Project for a Scientific Psychology*. *S. E., 1*: 281–391. London: Hogarth.

Gilligan, C. (1994). *La moral y la teoría. Psicología del desarrollo femenino*. México: Fondo de Cultura Económica.

Irigaray, L. (1984). *El cuerpo a cuerpo con la madre*. Madrid: Cátedra.

Irigaray, L. (1997). *Ser dos: bosquejo de una felicidad en la historia*. Buenos Aires: Paidós.

Klein, M. (1988). *Envy and Gratitude and Other Works 1946–1963*, M. M. R. Khan (Ed.). London: Hogarth Press.

Kristeva, J. (1993). *Las nuevas enfermedades del alma*. Madrid: Cátedra.

Lacan, J. (1983). El estadio del espejo como formador de la función del yo ["je"] tal como se nos revela en la experiencia psicoanalítica. In: *Escritos 1*. Mexico: Siglo veintiuno editores. [Original work published in 1949].

Levinas, E. (2000). *Ética e infito*. Madrid: A. Machado Libros, S.A.

Levinton, N. (2000). *El superyó femenino*: *La moral en las mujeres*. Madrid: Biblioteca Nueva.

Quinodoz, J. M. (1993). *La soledad domesticada*. Buenos Aires: Paidós.

INDEX

For Product Safety Concerns and Information please contact our EU
representative GPSR@taylorandfrancis.com
Taylor & Francis Verlag GmbH, Kaufingerstraße 24, 80331 München, Germany

www.ingramcontent.com/pod-product-compliance
Lightning Source LLC
Chambersburg PA
CBHW050449051126
54379CB00003B/71
9780367104184